MAMMOGRAPHY EXAM REVIEW

Deborah Phlipot, B.Ed., R.T.(R)
Instructor of Radiography
Lima Technical College
Lima, Ohio

Richard R. Carlton, M.S., R.T.(R)
Chairman of Radiography
Lima Technical College
Lima, Ohio

M. Judy McLaughlin, M.S., R.T.(R)
Division Chair, Biological Sciences Division
Lexington Community College
Lexington, Kentucky

Patricia A. Miller, B.H.S., R.T.(R)(M)
Instructor of Radiography
Lexington Community College
Lexington, Kentucky

Technical Sales Representative
Marmer X-Ray, Inc.
Cincinnati, Ohio

Mammography Specialist
Bennett X-Ray Corporation
Copiague, New York

J.B. Lippincott Company
Philadelphia

Acquisitions Editor: Andrew Allen
Production Manager: Virginia Barishek
Cover Designer: Tom Jackson
Printer/Binder: R. R. Donnelley & Sons Co.

10 9 8 7 6 5 4 3

ISBN 0-397-55019-7

Any procedure or practice described in this book should be applied by the health-care practitioner under appropriate supervision in accordance with professional standards of care used with regard to the unique circumstances that apply in each practice situation. Care has been taken to confirm the accuracy of information presented and to describe generally accepted practices. However, the authors, editors, and publisher cannot accept any responsibility for errors or omissions or for any consequences from application of the information in this book and make no warranty, express or implied, with respect to the contents of the book.

NWST
I AFG 3503

Figure 3 and 5 used with permission from Akesson, Elizabeth J., Loeb, Jacques, A., and Wilson-Pauwels, Linda. *Thompson's Core Textbook of Anatomy*, Philadelphia: J.B. Lippincott Co., 2nd ed., 1990.

Figure 7, 8, 9, and 10 used with permission from Andolina, V.F., Lille, S., Willison, K.M., *Mammographic Imaging: A Practical Guide*, Philadelphia: J.B. Lippincott, 1992.

ABOUT THE AUTHORS

Deborah Phlipot-Scroggins holds a certificate of advanced qualifications in mammography and cardiovascular - interventional technology from the ARRT and is Instructor of Radiography at The University of Texas-Galveston College. Deb has 14 years of experience in radiography and has taught for 4 years.

Richard R. Carlton is Chairman and Assistant Professor of Radiography at Lima Technical College in Lima, Ohio. He holds a certificate of advanced qualifications in cardiovascular - interventional technology from the ARRT, has taught radiography for 15 years, and is the co-author of *Principles of Radiographic Imaging* and *Introduction to Radiography and Patient Care*. His *Radiography Exam Review* was published by J.B. Lippincott in 1992. Rick is the editor of *Radiologic Science and Education*, the journal of the Association of Educators in Radiological Sciences (AERS), and *Seminars in Radiologic Technology*. He is a charter Fellow of AERS.

Rick and Deb are also the authors *Cardiovascular-Interventional Exam Review*, published by J.B. Lippincott in 1992 and are currently working on *Computed Tomography Exam Review* and *Magnetic Resonance Imaging Exam Review*, to be published by Lippincott in 1994.

Judy McLaughlin is Chair of the Biological Sciences Division and Associate Professor at Lexington Community College in Lexington, Kentucky. She serves on the American College of Radiology/Center for Disease Control cooperative committee to develop a mammography curriculum for radiologic technologists. Judy has also served on the American Cancer Society task force for mammography in Kentucky. She has taught for 14 years, including 12 as radiography program coordinator.

Patricia Miller holds a certificate of advanced qualifications in mammography from the ARRT and has 20 years of experience in radiography. She has been Technical Sales Representative and Mammography Specialists for 2 1/2 years. Pat is also Instructor of Radiography at Lexington Community College in Lexington, Kentucky.

Camera-ready copy produced by Linda Benson, Secretary I, Lima Technical College, Lima, Ohio.

to
my husband, Tom

to
the women in my life, Hazel, Lynn, and Michelle Carlton

to
my husband, John, and my children, Jennifer and Michael

to
my husband, Raymond, and my children

TABLE OF CONTENTS

* Question subject areas © 1991, The American Registry of Radiologic Technologists

PREFACE

This Mammography Exam Review is designed to assist persons preparing for the Mammography Advanced Level Examination of the American Registry of Radiologic Technologists (ARRT).

The American Registry of Radiologic Technologists does not review, evaluate, or endorse publications. Permission to reproduce ARRT copyrighted materials within this publication should not be construed as an endorsement of the publication by the ARRT. Any implication of ARRT approval of this book violates the policies of the ARRT. We have never served as a member of an ARRT mammography examination committee to review question items, nor have we had any questions accepted for consideration for the mammography examination. The questions in this book have not to our knowledge been used for any ARRT examination in radiography.

Although two new mammography texts for radiologic technologists are due for publication this year (see Andolina and Wentz in references), it has been difficult for educators to locate authoritative reference resources on mammography. Therefore, we have attempted to cite most of the current journal and physician references.

The reference citations are accurate enough to assist any medical librarian in obtaining the sources for anyone wishing to begin comprehensive study of any of the ARRT Mammography Examination content areas.

Every attempt has been made to provide example questions from the entire spectrum of mammographic procedures, especially information that appears in the most popular textbooks in current use. Because this is a new certification examination, everyone, educators and practitioners alike, will need time to adjust to the content necessary to be successful on this examination.

Although we have no special knowledge of the examination, we hope we have been able to compile a useful review of relevant subject content and hope it proves useful to those preparing for the examination. We welcome comments from users of this book, especially constructive criticism.

Deb Phlipot and Rick Carlton
Lima, Ohio
Judy McLaughlin and Pat Miller
Lexington, Kentucky

January 1992

ACKNOWLEDGEMENTS

This book went from concept to draft to publication in less than three months. Hopefully this is not overly obvious in the text. This was possible solely due to the confidence of Andrew Allen at Lippincott. We wish to thank Dennis Spragg and Andrew Shappell at Lima Tech for supporting us during the hectic weeks we were in production. Without their support we could not have taken the time to produce this work. Mary Kay Verhoff and Carole Cramer at St. Rita's Medical Center in Lima provided significant clinical insights which were greatly appreciated. This is Linda Benson's third book project for us and, as always, her patience and ability to produce the work was essential. Thanks to Roberta Miller at Medical College Hospital in Toledo, Ohio and to Margaret Botsco, R.T.(R), Mammography Consultant, Huntington Beach, CA, for their prompt and insightful critiques of the manuscript. Finally, the support of our authoring attempts by Sam Bassitt, our Vice President of Instruction at Lima Technical College, has given us the necessary tools to complete this project.

Rick Carlton and Deb Phlipot

Thanks, one more time, to my wife Lynn for her continuing patience and support for my authoring attempts.

Rick Carlton

Special thanks and appreciation to Rick for his confidence in my abilities and for inspiring me through the authoring process.

Deb Phlipot

I would like to acknowledge the following people for their help and guidance: Dr. Carol Stelling, Karen Duncan, Dr. Jerry Buchanan, Randie Hale, Jan Sonnanstine, Barbara Vieson, Leah Levine, John Ataman, and the other authors.

Patricia A. Miller

Finally, we all acknowledge the inspiration we have received from our students and from practicing mammographers everywhere. Your hard work and the exemplary care of your patients can now be professionally recognized through national certification. We wish you the very best of results on your examination.

TERMINOLOGY

It is the policy of the ARRT that new terminology and concepts will be used on examination questions only after they achieve general usage throughout the profession. The Twelfth International Congress of Anatomists in 1985 adopted substantial alterations of anatomical nomenclature that were subsequently published in the sixth edition of *Nomina Anatomica* in 1989. Although these alterations have very recently begun to appear in radiological literature, they were not used in this book as it will probably be some time before either the profession or the ARRT adopts them.

The American College of Radiology is in the process of establishing new positioning terminology for Mammography. Because it is not expected that the new terminology will be adopted by the ARRT or appear on the Mammography examination immediately, the questions in this book have retained the older terminology. Appendix E provides a guide to the anticipated new terminology.

USING THIS REVIEW TO BEST ADVANTAGE

This review is designed to be used as a helpful tool in reminding mammography technologists of content that was learned some time ago, diagnosing weak areas for further study, and adding a strong measure of confidence to those subject areas in which both academic and clinical success have already been proven.

This review is not a substitute for several years of practice in mammography. It is not possible to prepare for a major national certification examination by studying from questions. Instead it is critical to engage in the careful study of appropriate textbooks in radiologic technology, such as those listed in the reference section.

To use this review to best advantage it is suggested that study begin 2-3 months prior to the examination. This review can be used as a pre-test by taking one of the examinations (see <u>Directions For Answering Questions In This Book</u>), then reviewing references books, and finally taking another one of the examinations in this book as a post-test. A third examination from this book can serve as a double check or a mid-review assessment of progress.

Each question includes the answer, a short explanation, and references for further information. Answers to questions appear in three locations; at the edge of the page underneath the question, in the answer section with the explanation and reference at the end of the book, and in the answer keys to the simulated examinations at the end of the book.

Explanations and References
Short explanations are located at the end of the book in an attempt to keep the question pages uncluttered. The explanation is followed by a reference if further review or study is needed. The short phrases are the index words that should be used to locate more information in the index of any text. Several references that have information on the topic are then provided.

It is a good strategy to scan your favorite textbook in each major subject area, skimming headers, bold or italicized words, and figure captions. Most authors emphasize important content by using these devices to bring attention to a content area. Figures are expensive to produce and are used only when important ideas need to be explained carefully. Reading the figure captions is a good way to catch all the high points of a particular text. When something is not remembered, either because it has been forgotten or was never taught or learned previously, stop and study the section. If the entire textbook is reviewed in this manner, it assures students that few of the "nationally recognized" content areas have been overlooked. The table below illustrates common subject areas for which textbooks should be obtained for this approach to preparing for a certification examination.

COMMON SUBJECT AREAS FOR TEXTBOOK REVIEW
with recommended references
(full citations at end of book)

ANATOMY, PHYSIOLOGY, AND PATHOLOGY
Thibodeau
Ballinger
Hole
Laudicina

MAMMOGRAPHY
American College of Radiology
American Society of Radiologic Technologists
Anderson
Feig
NCRP Report No. 85

X-RAY TUBES, RADIOGRAPHIC PRINCIPLES OF EXPOSURE, FILM PROCESSING, AND FILM-SCREEN COMBINATIONS
Ballinger
Bushong
Carlton
Curry
Haus
Tabar

Simulated Examinations
This book is also designed to incorporate four full length simulated examinations. These examinations can be taken by paging through the book and answering the questions according to the large bold numbers that appear next to the binding side of each question. Answering all the examination 1 questions will provide 100 questions of a wide variety of content areas. Each examination can be graded by checking your answers against the simulated examination answer keys that make up appendix A, B, C, and D.

Appendix Table
A table of common abbreviations is included as Appendix E.

SUGGESTED STUDY REFERENCES

Ideally, all the books listed in the References section should be used in study. However, it is highly recommended that the mammography study guides published by the American College of Radiology (ACR) and the American Society of Radiologic Technologists (ASRT) be used as a base for study. The ACR guide is the *Mammography Quality Control Radiologic Technologist Manual* and the ASRT guide is *Fundamentals of Mammography: The Quest for Quality Positioning Guidebook.*

In addition, the National Council on Radiation Protection and Measurements' NCRP Report No. 85, *Mammography: A User's Guide* is highly recommended.

For anatomy, physiology, and pathology Ballinger's *Merrill's Atlas of Radiographic Positions and Radiologic Procedures* (Volume 3), a good basic anatomy and physiology text (such as Hole's *Human Anatomy and Physiology* or Thibodeau's *Anthony's Textbook of Anatomy and Physiology*), and a radiographic pathology text (such as Eisenberg's *Comprehensive Pathology for Radiologic Technologists*) are recommended.

It is also recommended that a basic x-ray equipment and principles of exposure and processing text be consulted (such as Carlton and Adler's *Principles of Radiographic Imaging*, Curry's *Christensen's Physics of Diagnostic Radiology*, or Bushong's *Radiologic Science for Technologists*).

All these references will be found in most medical libraries, radiologic technology faculty offices, hospital radiology departments, and radiologists' personal libraries.

SUGGESTED STUDY HABITS

This is an important test in your career. Do not underestimate your need to study for it. A minimum of a two month plan is necessary to prepare properly. A 2 or 3 week study plan is usually insufficient to permit proper coverage of the multiple content areas you must investigate in depth. Beginning more than 6 months before the examination is not advisable because your ability to maintain an effective level of concentration will be exhausted by the time you begin the critical 1-2 months prior to your test date.

Technologists who have been out of school for some time may need an additional period to get back into study habits. It is advisable to establish a written study schedule and adhere to it. Many students find that requiring double study time when a session is missed is the only way to maintain a regular schedule.

It is strongly recommended that every technologist obtain a copy of the content specifications, listing the outline of subjects to be examined. They appear in the *Examinee Handbook for Advanced Level Examinations*, (which also includes the application for examination), available from the ARRT at 1255 Northland Drive, Mendota Heights, Minnesota 55120, phone 612-687-0048. This document subdivides the number of questions in each content category by subject and is the best study guide. Its proper use permits students to concentrate on reviewing information in heavily weighted areas to gain maximum advantage from the probability of the content expected on the examination.

General Habits
1.   A quiet place away from distractions such as music and talking helps with concentration.

2.   Group study sessions are valuable but should be limited to 3-4 persons and should not be the only study method.

3.   Concentrate on a single topic area at one time (such as procedures-patient care or instrumentation).

4.   Areas of difficulty should be noted for further study by reading a different textbook, consulting with an instructor, or attending a review session.

Learning Skills

Remember that isolated data is difficult to remember. Try to use concepts to remember data instead of just memorizing the data.

When data must be memorized it is often helpful to use acronyms, such as those in the abbreviations and acronyms appendix. You can invent your own acronyms for data as well.

You can only remember so much information. Be selective in what you choose to memorize so that other more important knowledge is not lost in the process.

Students wishing to further improve their study habits may benefit from reading chapter 2 "Developing Thinking Skills" of the J.B. Lippincott book *Nurse's Guide to Successful Test-Taking* by Marian B. Sides and Nancy B. Cailles, 1989.

HELPFUL HINTS FOR TAKING
NATIONAL CERTIFICATION EXAMINATIONS

Take two calculators that are battery (not solar) powered. Include new batteries for both. Work a variety of different types of problems with both calculators to be sure you know how to use the keyboard before you leave for the examination site. Do not take a programmable calculator to the examination as you could be accused of cheating by entering formulas into the memory.

1. Always read every word of all instructions. There may be a slight change from your past experiences that could cause correct answers to be marked wrong.

2. Most questions are written with the distractors (the possible choices that are labeled a,b,c, and d) designed so there is a correct answer, a closely related choice, and two choices that are less likely. Consequently the best method of answering all questions is:

    (1) Read the entire question and all choices before choosing an answer. Although the first choice may appear correct, the fourth choice may turn out to be a better or more comprehensive answer.

    (2) Look for key words that target important information and don't assume information unless it is stated.

    (3) Determine which two choices are the less likely ones and eliminate them first.

(4)   Choose the best answer from the two remaining choices. When you must guess, this process improves the odds of guessing a correct answer from 25% to 50%. If you guess at 20 questions over the entire examination, this produces 10 correct answers instead of only 5. This is enough to raise your entire examination score by 5 percentile points!

3.   Always work all mathematical calculations twice to make sure you didn't press the wrong key by mistake.

4.   Do not spend a long period (more than 2-3 minutes) on a single question. You can mark it and return after you have completed the entire examination. It is normal to have numerous questions that require more than 2-3 minutes. Nearly all students will return to re-study particularly difficult questions after all the questions have been attempted once.

5.   It is acceptable to skip difficult questions entirely and return to them after completing the entire examination.

6.   At question number 50 remember to check the time and see how you are progressing. If you have taken longer than 1 1/2 hours to reach question 50 you must work faster. If this is the case, when you reach number 75 check the time again and if necessary, mark in guesses for all questions on the answer card. Then continue the examination by erasing the guess and entering your answer. In this manner, if time is called while you are working you will have 25% of the questions you did not answer marked correctly just because of your guesses. These extra correct answers could make the difference between passing and failing the examination.

7.   After completion the entire examination should be read a second time to search for errors in marking answers.

8.   When re-reading the examination remember that the first choice of an answer has the highest probability of being correct. However, if you can determine that you didn't read the question correctly, or if you have obtained more information from answering other questions, don't hesitate to change an answer.

9.   Always mark an answer for all questions, even if it is a guess. With 4 distractors, 25% of all guesses will be correct and these add to your total score. For example, if you only knew the answers to 80 of the 100 questions and you answered 73 (73%) correctly, there is a possibility that you would not pass the examination. However, if you guessed at all 20 of the questions you did not know, it is highly likely that you would get 5 more questions right, raise your total score to 78%, probably pass the examination, and become a certified mammography technologist.

Technologists may benefit from the excellent discussion on taking tests in chapter 4 "Strategies for Effective Test-Taking" of the J.B. Lippincott book *Nurse's Guide to Successful Test-Taking* by Marian B. Sides and Nancy B. Cailles, 1989.

DIRECTIONS FOR ANSWERING THE QUESTIONS
IN THIS BOOK

Select the single best answer for each question from the four possible answers or completions.

Answers

The answer to each question is printed at the edge of the page underneath the question. Lifting the page slightly will reveal the answer. (Each answer has its question number in superscript to avoid mixups.)

Answers, Explanations, and References

The Answers and Explanations section at the end of the book gives the answer again with a short explanation. Each explanation is followed in bold type by the index keywords and references necessary to locate a full discussion of the content in the question. The complete library citation for each reference is listed in the References section at the end of the book.

Simulated Examinations

Four complete simulated examinations are possible by answering the questions according to the large bold numbers on the binding side of each question. The question number for each simulated examination appears as a superscript to the examination number. Answer keys to the Four simulated examinations appear in the appendices.

Examples

The answers to questions E1-E4 appear by slightly lifting the page to show them underneath. Each answer has its question number as a superscript to avoid confusion.

To take the simulated examinations, question E1 would be the first question in simulated examination 1 while question E2 would be the second. The next question in simulated examination 1 would be question E4 (which is the third question in examination 1).

┌─ Simulated Exam   Question # ─┐
│ ┌─ Question #   Answer ┐│
↓ ↓   ↓ ↓

1^1 E1.   What is mammography?

          a. radiographic examination of the mammary ducts
          b. radiographic examination of the chest
          c. radiographic examination of the breast
          d. the study of gynecological pathology

1^2 E2.   Which of the following are part of the breast?

          1. nipple
          2. areola
          3. inframammary crease

          a. 1 and 2 only
          b. 1 and 3 only
          c. 2 and 3 only
          d. 1, 2, & 3

2^1 E3.   What do the initials BSE represent?

          a. breast self examination
          b. base standard extrapolation
          c. breast size examination
          d. benign screening examination

1^3 E4.   What term describes a breast cancer?

          a. benign
          b. malignant
          c. Osteod's tumor
          d. sarcoma

Patient Education

B ^{5}

B ^{6}

A ^{7}

1^1 1.   The breasts of women exposed to radiation after the age of 35 are:

    a.   less sensitive to radiation
    b.   more sensitive to higher doses
    c.   more sensitive to lower doses
    d.   this risk is not age related

1^2 2.   The incidence of naturally occurring breast cancers: C[E1]

    a.   increases after age 50
    b.   decreases after age 50
    c.   doubles between age 40-50
    d.   reduces by half between age 40-50

2^1 3.   Which of the following are not one of the four main sources of epidemiological data on the breast?   D[E2]

    a.   Japanese atomic bomb survivors
    b.   shoe store fluoroscopy operators
    c.   benign breast disease patients
    d.   tuberculosis patients

2^2 4.   Factors that increase the risk factor for breast cancer do not include: A[E3]

    a.   first pregnancy after 30
    b.   post menopause
        estrogen replacement therapy
    c.   early menarche and late menopause   B[E4]
    d.   family history of breast cancer

Patient Education

5. Which of the following populations are more prone to risk of breast cancer?

3^1

    a. Asians
    b. Americans and Canadians
    c. Mexicans
    d. Japanese

A^{11} 6. The carcinogenic effect of ionizing radiation on the breast:

3^2

    1. has a latency period of 7-10 years
    2. is genetically linked
    3. persists for the patient's lifetime

B^{12}
    a. 1 and 2 only
    b. 1 and 3 only
    c. 2 and 3 only
    d. 1, 2, & 3

7. Which of the following dietary factors do not appear to increase the risk of breast cancer?

4^1

C^{13}
    a. high caloric intake
    b. high fat content
    c. high protein content
    d. above average alcohol consumption

4^2 8. Which type factors have not been shown to have a significant effect on the risk of developing breast cancer?

   a. personal
   b. environmental
   c. economic
   d. educational level

A ^{1}

1^3 9. According to the American Cancer Society guidelines for mammography, when should the baseline mammogram be performed?

   a. between age 25-30
   b. between age 35-40
   c. between age 45-50
   d. after menopause

C ^{2}

2^3 10. According to the American Cancer Society guidelines for mammography, a woman between the ages of 40 and 49 should undergo mammographic examination every:

   a. 6-9 months
   b. 1-2 years
   c. 3-4 years
   d. 5 years

B ^{3}

B ^{4}

Patient Education

11. How often do the American Cancer Society guidelines for mammography recommend mammographic examination for a woman over the age of 50?

3^3

    a.   annually
    b.   every 2 years
    c.   every 5 years
    d.   whenever abnormal changes are noted

A[18]

12. How often should breast self-examination be done by postmenopausal women?

4^3

    a.   weekly
    b.   monthly
    c.   every 6 months
    d.   annually

B[19]

13. In which area is the highest incidence of breast cancer found?

1^4

    a.   behind the nipple
    b.   areola
    c.   upper outer quadrant
    d.   upper inner quadrant

A[20]

1^5 14.   Which of the following is/are the most common sign/s of breast cancer?
1.   swelling
2.   nipple discharges
3.   lumps or thickening

a.   1 only
b.   2 only
c.   3 only
d.   1, 2, & 3

D ^{8}

1^6 15.   What is the approximate skin thickness of a normal breast?

a.   0.05 mm
b.   0.5 mm
c.   1.5 mm
d.   3.0 mm

B ^{9}

2^4 16.   Which term defines lactation unrelated to pregnancy?

a.   galactorrhea
b.   adenosis
c.   papillomatosis
d.   galactocele

B ^{10}

2^5 17.   Which of the following structures is involved with skin retraction?

a.   lactiferous sinuses
b.   nipple
c.   areola
d.   suspensory ligaments (ligaments of Cooper)

18. Which of the following would be considered a skin retraction? **2**⁶

1. small local dimpling
2. shrinkage of the entire breast
3. single dilated duct

a. 1 and 2 only
b. 1 and 3 only
c. 2 and 3 only
d. 1, 2, & 3

A ²⁴

19. Which of the following is a leading cause of cancer mortality in females of all ages? **3**⁴

a. colon
b. breast
c. lung
d. skin

20. Which of the following defines a cystic dilation of one of the major ducts of the mammary gland? **3**⁵

D ²⁵

1. galactocele
2. duct papilloma
3. fibroadenoma

a. 1 only
b. 2 only
c. 3 only
d. 1, 2, & 3

C ²⁶

3⁶   21.   Which of the following types of breast carcinoma has the highest incidence?

    a.   intraductal
    b.   invasive
    c.   lobular
    d.   lipoma

4⁴   22.   Approximately what percentage of women have breast cysts?   C [14]

    a.   < 5%
    b.   10%
    c.   25%
    d.   > 50%

4⁵   23.   Which of the following are potential post breast surgery complications?   C [15]

    a.   lymphedema, and arm stiffness
    b.   uticaria and lymphedema
    c.   subdural hematoma
            and hepatomegaly
    d.   diaphragmatic rupture

A [16]

D [17]

Patient Education

24. Which of the following are valid indications for adjuvant radiotherapy?

4^6

1. 5 cm tumor site
2. 20% positive axillary lymph nodes
3. small medially located tumor

a. extended laterally
b. flexed medially
A [30]   c. 2 and 3
d. 1, 2, & 3

25. Which of the following determines possible radiation risk to the patient from mammography?

1^7

1. mean glandular dose
2. patient age at initial examination
3. patient age at follow up examination

a. 1 only
b. 2 only
C [34]   c. 3 only
d. 1, 2, & 3

26. Which is the approximate average glandular dose for a screening mammogram?

1^8

a. grid biased x-ray tube
b. high frequency generator
c. beam splitting mirror
d. roll film camera
D [32]

2⁷   27.   Which of the following variables affect breast dose per projection?

1.   degree of breast compression
2.   breast size and adiposity   A²¹
3.   beam HVL energy

a.   1 and 2 only
b.   1 and 3 only
c.   2 and 3 only
d.   1, 2, & 3

2⁸   28.   What is the current state of the incidence of breast cancer for American females?   D²²

a.   decreasing slowly
b.   decreasing rapidly
c.   increasing slowly
d.   remaining the same

3⁷   29.   Which of the following is not a factor that increases the risk of breast cancer for women?   A²³

a.   obesity
b.   pregnancy after age 30
c.   family history of breast cancer
d.   living in urban areas

30. Which of the following factors increases the incidence of breast cancer in American women?

3⁸

1. affluence
2. fat content of diet
3. number of children after the first one

C³⁷

a. 1 and 2 only
b. 1 and 3 only
c. 2 and 3 only
d. 1, 2, & 3

31. Which of the following variables is not true regarding the treatment of breast cancer?

4⁷

a. it is more aggressive in younger women
b. older women are more prone to the disease

D³⁸

c. low white blood cell counts increase survival rates
d. a high fat content diet increases the risk of the disease

32. Approximately what percentage of patients diagnosed with breast cancer exhibit none of the known risk factors?

4⁸

a. 40%
b. 50%
c. 60%
d. 70%

D³⁹

1⁹ 33. The American Cancer Society recommends a monthly breast self examination beginning at what age?

    a.   20
    b.   25
    c.   35
    d.   40

1¹⁰ 34. The importance of breast self examination is stressed partly due to the fact that mammography will miss what percentage of all cancers?   D²⁷

    a.   1-2%
    b.   5-7%
    c.   10-15%
    d.   40-50%

1¹¹ 35. Using the flats of which digits produce the best breast self examination technique?   C²⁸

    a.   thumb and 1st finger
    b.   1st, 2nd, and 3rd fingers
    c.   2nd, 3rd, and 4th fingers
    d.   3rd and 4th fingers

2⁹ 36. Which of the following is the most effective method of teaching breast self examination?   D²⁹

    a.   observing a physician demonstration
    b.   practicing on a life-like model
    c.   reading a pamphlet
    d.   viewing a videotape

Patient Education

37. What position of the arm best accomplishes a
     breast self examination of the tail of Spence?

2^{10}

    a.   extended laterally
    b.   flexed medially
    c.   raised over the head
    d.   posteriorly and inferiorly flexed

D [43]

38. Which of the following methods of breast self
     examination are acceptable?

2^{11}

    1.   vertical strip
    2.   spiral
    3.   quadrant by quadrant

A [44]

    a.   1 and 2 only
    b.   1 and 3 only
    c.   2 and 3 only
    d.   1, 2, & 3

39. Which of the following are valid arguments
     against breast self examination?

3^{9}

    1.   enhances the risk of future invasive
         studies
    2.   compliance is best from the age group
         least likely to develop cancer
    3.   self discovered lesions are 80-90%

D [45]   benign

    a.   1 and 2 only
    b.   1 and 3 only
    c.   2 and 3 only
    d.   1, 2, & 3

24

3[10]   40.   Which of the following is an advantage to teaching breast self examination with a screening program?

a.   interval cancers may be detected
b.   cost of screening procedures is lowered
c.   overall cancer survival rates will increase
d.   patient compliance will decrease

A [33]

3[11]   41.   What is the best time after the onset of menstruation to perform a breast self examination?

a.   1-2 days
b.   7-10 days
c.   15-20 days
d.   28-30 days

C [34]

4[9]   42.   What should be the position of the patient's arms during the visual inspection as part of a breast self examination or a clinical examination?

C [35]

a.   semi-pronated
b.   extended laterally
c.   elbow flexed with forearm across abdomen
d.   elbows flexed, hands behind head, with elbows as posterior as possible

B [36]

43. Which of the following is not a shortcoming of breast self examination screening? **4**[10]

   a.   it is inferior to a professional examination
   b.   it is inferior to mammography
   c.   it produces primarily benign lesions
   d.   delays in physician visits often result

B[49] 44. Which of the following is a potential disadvantage of breast self examination? **4**[11]

   a.   inaccuracy
   b.   low cost
   c.   can be done in private at home
   d.   has a low pain threshold

A[50] 45. Which of the following is true regarding ultrasonographic examination of the breast? **1**[12]

   1.   distinguishes benign from malignant lesions
   2.   avoids the use of ionizing radiation
   3.   is painless

C[51]
   a.   1 and 2 only
   b.   1 and 3 only
   c.   2 and 3 only
   d.   1, 2, & 3

1[13]   46.   Which of the following is not true regarding a wide needle breast biopsy?

a.   a cutting core needle is used
b.   a local anesthetic
c.   can be an outpatient procedure
d.   is relatively painless

1[14]   47.   Galactography is useful in diagnosing: A[40]

1.   intraductal masses
2.   intraductal papillomas
3.   occult carcinomas

a.   1 and 2 only
b.   1 and 3 only
c.   2 and 3 only   B[41]
d.   1, 2, & 3

2[12]   48.   Which of the following is not a valid use of ultrasonography of the breast?

a.   evaluation of multiple cysts
b.   tumor detection
c.   differentiation between cysts and solid masses
d.   screening examinations for fatty breasts

D[42]

49. Which of the following is not a purpose of a hole plate during a breast needle biopsy? **2**¹³

C⁵⁵

    a.   to compress the breast
    b.   establish a sterile field
    c.   to provide a grid reference for guidance of the needle
    d.   to provide a visual reference for needle localization on the mammographic image

50. Which of the following is a valid use of pneumocystography? **2**¹⁴

    a.   cyst treatment
    b.   cyst diagnosis
    c.   cyst localization
    d.   tumor detection

D⁵⁶ 51. Which of the following is injected through the blunt tip of the needle during galactography? **3**¹²

    a.   oil based contrast media
    b.   methylene blue
    c.   water based contrast media
    d.   air

3[13]   52.   Which of the following radiographic procedures is most similar to galactography?

    a.   bronchography
    b.   angiography
    c.   coronary catheterization
    d.   discography

D[46]

3[14]   53.   Which of the following are true about various dedicated breast ultrasonographic units?

    1.   patients can be examined prone
    2.   patients can be examined supine
    3.   only sagittal plane images can be produced

    a.   1 and 2 only
    b.   1 and 3 only
    c.   2 and 3 only
    d.   1, 2, & 3

D[47]

4[12]   54.   Which of the following are true regarding surgical breast biopsy?

    1.   confirms needle biopsy results
    2.   provides conclusive diagnosis
    3.   produces about 75% benign diagnosis

    a.   1 only
    b.   2 only
    c.   3 only
    d.   1, 2, & 3

D[48]

55.　What is the primary purpose of a breast biopsy?　**4**¹³

    a.　cyst detection
    b.　tumor size evaluation
    c.　occult lesion detection
    d.　tumor contrast enhancement

56.　Which of the following can be diagnosed via galactography when evaluating nipple discharge?　**4**¹⁴

    1.　duct ectasia
    2.　endocrine changes
    3.　fibrocystic changes

    a.　1 and 2 only
    b.　1 and 3 only
    c.　2 and 3 only
    d.　1, 2, & 3

B ⁵⁹

C ⁶⁰

Clinical Breast Examination

1¹⁵   57.   In which quadrant of the breast is carcinoma least likely to develop?

     a.   UOQ
     b.   UIQ
     c.   LOQ
     d.   LIQ

A [52]

1¹⁶   58.   What terms can be used to describe the location of a lesion in the breast?

     a.   hours on a clock face
     b.   quadrants of the thorax
     c.   regions of the chest
     d.   cm from the sternoclavicular joints

A [53]

D [54]

Clinical Breast Examination

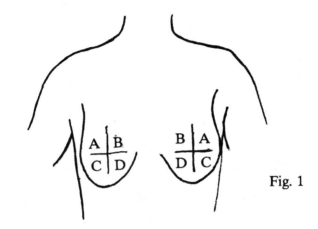

Fig. 1

D ⁶⁴

59. Which quadrant on the left breast represents
     a breast lesion determined to be in the 10
     o'clock position in Figure 1?

     2¹⁵

C ⁶⁵

     a.   A
     b.   B
     c.   C
     d.   D

60. Which quadrant could include a breast lesion
     determined to be in the 2 o'clock position in
     Figure 1?

     2¹⁶

B ⁶⁶

     1.   D
     2.   A
     3.   B

     a.   1 and 2 only
     b.   1 and 3 only
     c.   2 and 3 only
     d.   1, 2, & 3

3¹⁵   61.   Which quadrant includes a right breast lesion determined to be in the 2 o'clock position in Figure 1?

     a.   A
     b.   B
     c.   C
     d.   D

D [57]

3¹⁶   62.   Which quadrant would include a left breast lesion determined to be in the 8 o'clock position?

     a.   UIQ
     b.   UOQ
     c.   LIQ
     d.   LOQ

A [58]

4¹⁵   63.   Which of the following factors determine the incidence of occurrence of cancer in various quadrants?

     1.   endocrine presence
     2.   quantity of glandular tissue
     3.   family history of location

     a.   1 only
     b.   2 only
     c.   3 only
     d.   1, 2, & 3

Clinical Breast Examination

64. If a lesion is localized at 5 o'clock on the right breast, in which quadrant would the lesion be located?

4^{16}

    a. UOQ
    b. UIQ
    c. LOQ
    d. LIQ

C [70]

65. Which of the following is not necessary during the visual inspection of the patient prior to mammography?

1^{17}

    a. all jewelry has been removed from the neck and torso
    b. a strong light is used
    c. all deodorant is removed
    d. both seated and recumbent examination

C [71]

66. Which of the following should be noted as part of the visual breast examination?

1^{18}

    a. clavicular-nipple distance
    b. areolar size
    c. nipple length
    d. areolae color

A [72]

2[17] 67. Which of the following lymph node signs does not require further evaluation?

    a.   0.5 cm
    b.   1.5 cm
    c.   fixed nodes
    d.   hard nodes

2[18] 68. Which of the following are unacceptable immediately prior to mammography?   B [61]

    1.   talcum powder
    2.   deodorant
    3.   high fat content foods

    a.   1 and 2 only   C [62]
    b.   1 and 3 only
    c.   2 and 3 only
    d.   1, 2, & 3

3[17] 69. Which of the following anatomical anomalies should be noted during a physical breast examination?

    1.   supernummary nipples
    2.   aplasia
    3.   nipple inversion

    a.   1 and 2 only   B [63]
    b.   1 and 3 only
    c.   2 and 3 only
    d.   1, 2, & 3

70. Which of the following is the primary reason it is important to note the location of skin moles on the breast?

3[18]

a. it may simulate a benign cyst
b. it can superimpose micro-calcifications
c. it can simulate a well circumscribed intermammary lesion

D[76]

d. the scatter it produces may obscure other lesions

71. Which of the following is a potential artifact appearance of a recent surgical scar?

4[17]

a. malignant lesion
b. benign lesion
c. radial spiculations
d. benign cyst

A[77]

72. Which of the following are reasons why deodorants should be removed prior to mammographic examination?

4[18]

1. residues can appear radiopaque
2. residues can mimic micro-calcifications
3. fumes can begin premature film developing

B[78]

a. 1 and 2 only
b. 1 and 3 only
c. 2 and 3 only
d. 1, 2, & 3

1¹⁹ 73.   What is the proper position of the arms for breast and lymph node palpation during clinical examination?

   a.   semi-supinated at the sides
   b.   extended from the sides   A [67]
   c.   hands on hips with breasts thrust forward
   d.   hands locked behind head

1²⁰ 74.   Which of the following is part of the purpose of the technologist's physical examination of the breast?

   1.   making medical diagnosis
   2.   part of the screening examination
   3.   supplement the clinical history

                                                   A [68]
   a.   1 only
   b.   2 only
   c.   3 only
   d.   1, 2, & 3

2¹⁹ 75.   When performing an examination of the right breast, where should the technologist stand?

   a.   in front of the patient
   b.   behind the patient
   c.   at the patient's right side
   d.   at the patient's left side   D [69]

76. The visual inspection criteria for breast examination includes noting the following signs: 2^{20}

 1. scars
 2. moles
 3. lumps

 a. 1 and 2 only
 b. 1 and 3 only
D ^{81} c. 2 and 3 only
 d. 1, 2, & 3

77. What is the best position of the patient for palpation of the lymph nodes that drain the breast area? 3^{19}

 a. erect and bent forward at the waist
 b. erect and bent backward at the waist
 c. supine
 d. prone

D ^{82} 78. For which of the following is variable finger pressure valuable during breast physical examination? 3^{20}

 a. superficial lesions
 b. deep lesions
 c. malignant lesions
 d. cysts

B ^{83}

4[19]   79.   Which of the following become more prominent when the breast is examined with the hands behind the head?

1.   areas of retraction
2.   inverted nipples
3.   deviated nipples

C[73]

a.   1 and 2 only
b.   1 and 3 only
c.   2 and 3 only
d.   1, 2, & 3

4[20]   80.   What is the recommended method to obtain a view of the underside of heavy pendulous breasts?

a.   have the patient lift them
b.   have the patient bend to the affected side
c.   manually lift them
d.   manually push them to one side, then the other

C[74]

C[75]

81. Which of the following should influence the length of the interval between screening examinations of asymptomatic patients?

1²¹

1. density of breast parenchyma
2. age of the patient
B ⁸⁷ 3. positive family history

a. 1 and 2 only
b. 1 and 3 only
c. 2 and 3 only
d. 1, 2, & 3

82. Which of the following are causes of nipple discharge?

1²²

1. hypothalamic pituitary dysfunction
2. cystic change
3. oral contraceptives
B ⁸⁸

a. 1 only
b. 2 only
c. 3 only
d. 1, 2, & 3

83. During a mammographic evaluation the radiographer does not have a responsibility to:

1²³

C ⁸⁹

a. obtain a high quality examination
b. educate the patient on how to perform a breast self examination
c. reduce the anxiety level of the patient
d. coordinate clinical history with the radiologist

2²¹   84.   Which of the following are characteristic of fibroadenomas?

1.   micro-calcifications
2.   lobulated
3.   smooth margins

a.   1 and 2 only
b.   1 and 3 only
c.   2 and 3 only
d.   1, 2, & 3

D ⁷⁹

2²²   85.   Which of the following are valid methods for a patient to convey consent for an examination?

1.   written
2.   oral
3.   implied

a.   1 only
b.   2 only
c.   3 only
d.   1, 2, & 3

C ⁸⁰

2²³   86.   Which of the following is a common site for first re-occurrence of breast cancer?

a.   chest wall
b.   brain
c.   liver
d.   kidneys

┌─ Answer
│ ┌─ Question #
↓ ↓

Question # ─┐
Simulated Exam ─┐│
↓ ↓

87.   Women whose mothers or sisters have had premenopausal breast cancer have how many times the risk of developing the disease?

3^{21}

a.   same
b.   2-3
c.   4
d.   5

A^{92} 88.   Parity is important because increased risk of breast cancer has been shown in:

3^{22}

1.   females with live births prior to age 20
2.   childless females over age 30
3.   women with more than 3 children

a.   1 only
b.   2 only
c.   3 only
d.   1, 2, & 3

89.   Which of the following factors have been identified as risks for breast cancer?

3^{23}

a.   early menarche, early menopause
b.   late menarche, late menopause
c.   early menarche, late menopause
d.   late menarche, early menopause

4^{21} 90.   Which of the following visual changes are critical during the clinical history for mammography?

1.   size
2.   shape
3.   contour

a.   1 only
b.   2 only
c.   3 only
d.   1, 2, & 3

C [84]

4^{22} 91.   Which of the following is appropriate for a patient who reports nipple discharge?

1.   the breast should be milked
2.   a breast pump should be utilized
3.   a pathology sample should be obtained

a.   1 and 2 only
b.   1 and 3 only
c.   2 and 3 only
d.   1, 2, & 3

D [85]

A [86]

92. Which of the following is true regarding withdrawal of consent to perform mammography?

4^{23}

  a. it can be withdrawn verbally at any time

D⁹⁶

  b. it can be withdrawn verbally only in advance of the examination
  c. it can be withdrawn only in writing
  d. it can be withdrawn only with the prescribing physician's knowledge

D⁹⁷

B⁹⁸

Instrumentation

1²⁴   93.   What is the appropriate force for compression of the breast?

    a.   5-20 pounds
    b.   25-40 pounds
    c.   45-60 pounds
    d.   65-80 pounds

1²⁵   94.   What result does the anode-heel effect produce?

D [90]

    1.   greater image density toward the anode
    2.   less radiation intensity toward the cathode
    3.   greater radiation exposure toward the cathode

    a.   1 only
    b.   2 only
    c.   3 only
    d.   1, 2, & 3

1²⁶   95.   Which of the following is the most common factor affecting image quality in mammography?

D [91]

    a.   improperly applied compression
    b.   developer replenishment
    c.   grid selection
    d.   focal spot size

Instrumentation

96.   Which of the following are not recommended as a quarterly quality control test of mammographic equipment?   **1**²⁷

    a.   kVp accuracy
    b.   linearity
    c.   reproduceability
    d.   timer accuracy

B ¹⁰²   97.   Mammographic grids should have a minimum of how many lines per inch?   **1**²⁸

    a.   20
    b.   40
    c.   65
    d.   80

98.   Which of the following must be a consideration with a steep anode angle x-ray tube?   **1**²⁹

C ¹⁰³

    1.   the size of the primary beam field can be reduced
    2.   ion chamber sensitivity can be reduced
    3.   resolution can be increased

    a.   1 and 2 only
A ¹⁰⁴   b.   1 and 3 only
    c.   2 and 3 only
    d.   1, 2, & 3

1^{30} 99.   Which of the following focal spot sizes are within the range appropriate for standard mammographic examinations?

   a.   0.01 - 0.02 mm
   b.   0.1 - 0.2 mm
   c.   0.3 - 0.6 mm
   d.   1.2 - 1.5 mm

B ^{93}

1^{31} 100.   Which of the following are factors that account for the amount of compression obtained during mammography?

   1.   the degree of compressibility of the breast
   2.   patient tolerance
   3.   pathology

   a.   1 and 2 only
   b.   1 and 3 only
   c.   2 and 3 only
   d.   1, 2, & 3

C ^{94}

1^{32} 101.   Which of the following x-ray interactions produce photons that assist in producing optimal mammographic images?

   1.   Compton scatter
   2.   characteristic scatter
   3.   photoelectric scatter

   a.   1 and 2 only
   b.   1 and 3 only
   c.   2 and 3 only
   d.   1, 2, & 3

A ^{95}

102. Which of the following defines inherent filtration? **1**[33]

    a.   the filtration added to the primary beam

    b.   the filtration that is part of the structure of the x-ray tube

    c.   filtration added to compensate for differences in tissue composition

    d.   the total of the added and structural filtration

103. Which of the following devices can effectively accomplish quality control measurement of the compression device on a dedicated mammography unit? **2**[24]

    a.   tire pressure gauge

    b.   amperage compensator

A[108]   c.   bathroom scale

    d.   high voltage analyzer

104. What is the appropriate amount of molybdenum filtration that must be added to the inherent filtration of a mammography tube? **2**[25]

    a.   0.03 mm

    b.   0.30 mm

B[109]   c.   3.00 mm

    d.   30.0 mm

2^{26} 105. Which types of beam restriction devices can be used with a dedicated mammography unit?

1. aperture diaphragm
2. cylinder cone
3. collimator

C^{99}

a. 1 only
b. 2 only
c. 3 only
d. 1, 2, & 3

2^{27} 106. What is the recommended range of focal-film distances for mammography?

a. 25-35 cm (10-14")
b. 40-50 cm (16-20")
c. 55-65 cm (22-26")
d. 90-100 cm (36-40")

2^{28} 107. What terms are used to describe the piece of equipment that accomplishes breast compression?

D^{100}

1. plate
2. paddle
3. device

a. 1 only
b. 2 only
c. 3 only
d. 1, 2, & 3

C^{101}

Instrumentation

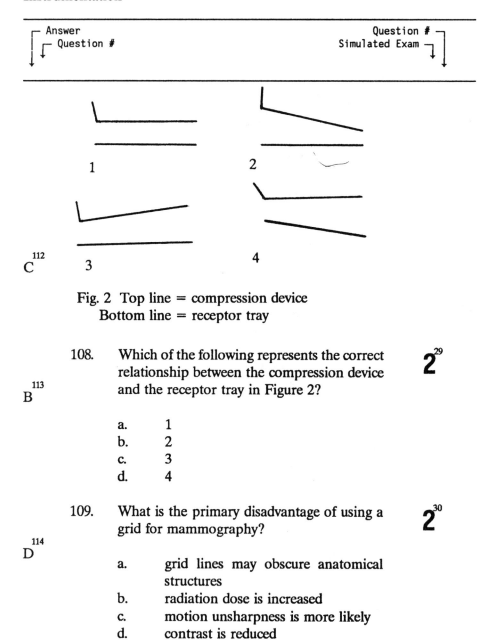

Fig. 2 Top line = compression device
Bottom line = receptor tray

108. Which of the following represents the correct relationship between the compression device and the receptor tray in Figure 2?

2^{29}

   a.   1
   b.   2
   c.   3
   d.   4

109. What is the primary disadvantage of using a grid for mammography?

2^{30}

   a.   grid lines may obscure anatomical structures
   b.   radiation dose is increased
   c.   motion unsharpness is more likely
   d.   contrast is reduced

112
C

113
B

114
D

2^{31} 110. Which of the following are differences between mammographic cassette film-screen tests and the film-screen tests used for diagnostic radiographic cassettes?

    1.   a finer wire mesh
    2.   lower kVp
    3.   a higher ratio grid

    a.   1 and 2 only
    b.   1 and 3 only
    c.   2 and 3 only
    d.   1, 2, & 3

105
D

2^{32} 111. Which of the following are reasons for using molybdenum in mammography tube targets?

    1.   it produces lower characteristic energy photons
    2.   it has a relatively low melting point
    3.   it emits a relatively uniform range of photon energies

106
C

    a.   1 and 2 only
    b.   1 and 3 only
    c.   2 and 3 only
    d.   1, 2, & 3

107
D

112. Which of the following is the proper relationship between the posterior edge of the compression plate and the body? **2**^{33}

    a. curved parallel to the chest wall
    b. angled posteriorly to the superior breast wall
    c. 90° to the chest wall
    d. angled to maximize patient comfort

113. Which of the following characteristic photons are within the range of molybdenum emissions? **3**^{24}

C ^{117}

    a. 7-10 keV
    b. 17-20 keV
    c. 20-35 keV
    d. 35-40 keV

114. What type of compression plate is recommended to uniformly reduce the entire breast thickness? **3**^{25}

B ^{118}

    a. sloping
    b. rounded
    c. angled
    d. right angle

D ^{119}

3²⁶ 115. Which of the following are limited by the heat unit rating of the mammographic x-ray tube?

1. kVp
2. mA
3. focal-film distance

a. 1 and 2 only
b. 1 and 3 only
c. 2 and 3 only
d. 1, 2, & 3

A ¹¹⁰

3²⁷ 116. Which of the following tube and film motions are commonly available with a dedicated mammography unit in order to adapt the unit to variations in patient body habitus?

1. raising and lowering
2. sagittal tomography
3. angling rotation (medial-lateral)

a. 1 and 2 only
b. 1 and 3 only
c. 2 and 3 only
d. 1, 2, & 3

B ¹¹¹

117. What is the most common relationship between the cathode-anode axis of the mammographic x-ray tube and the patient when the patient is facing the unit with the coronal plane at a right angle and the transverse plane parallel to the surface of the film?

3^{28}

123
B

1. parallel to the coronal plane
2. parallel to the transverse plane
3. parallel to the sagittal plane

a. 1 and 2 only
b. 1 and 3 only
c. 2 and 3 only
d. 1, 2, & 3

118. What is the K edge absorption of a molybdenum filter?

3^{29}

124
B

a. 14 keV
b. 20 keV
c. 68 keV
d. 74 keV

119. What grid ratio is recommended for mammography?

3^{30}

a. 16:1
b. 12:1
c. 8:1
d. 5:1

125
D

3³¹   120.   Which of the following statements are true?

1.   compression decreases variation in radiographic density of the breast
2.   compression increases separation of breast tissue
3.   compression increases geometric sharpness

a.   1 and 2 only
b.   1 and 3 only   115
c.   2 and 3 only   A
d.   1, 2, & 3

3³²   121.   Which of the following materials are recommended as the major mammography x-ray tube target material?

a.   molybdenum
b.   tungsten
c.   rhenium
d.   graphite

3³³   122.   Which of the following focal spot sizes are within the range appropriate for magnification mammography examinations?

116
B

a.   0.01 - 0.02 mm
b.   0.1 - 0.2 mm
c.   0.3 - 0.6 mm
d.   1.2 - 1.5 mm

123.   What is the primary characteristic of the manual compression control as compared to the foot pedal control on a dedicated mammography unit?

4²⁴

    a.   course adjustment
    b.   fine adjustment
    c.   lateral displacement
    d.   medial displacement

124.   Which of the following are acceptable focal spot measurement devices?

4²⁵

128
A

    1.   star test pattern
    2.   dosimeter
    3.   pinhole camera

    a.   1 and 2 only
    b.   1 and 3 only
    c.   2 and 3 only
    d.   1, 2, & 3

129
B

125.   Which of the following is a desirable characteristic of a compression device?

4²⁶

    1.   straight edge along the patient surface
    2.   foot pedal operation
    3.   automatic release upon exposure completion

130
B

    a.   1 only
    b.   2 only
    c.   3 only
    d.   1, 2, & 3

┌─ Simulated Exam   Question # ─┐
│ ┌─ Question #   Answer ┐ │
↓ ↓   ↓ ↓

4^{27} 126.   Which of the following describes the physical area of the focal spot that is impacted by the electrons from the x-ray tube filament?

         a.   effective focal spot
         b.   actual focal spot
         c.   hypothetical focal spot
         d.   focal track

4^{28} 127.   Which of the following statements is/are true regarding compression?   D [120]

         1.   it decreases patient radiation dose
         2.   it decreases image contrast
         3.   it decreases image resolution

         a.   1 only
         b.   2 only
         c.   3 only   A [121]
         d.   1, 2, & 3

B [122]

128. Which of the following are valid reasons for not using a standard diagnostic radiographic unit for mammography? **4**²⁹

134
A

1. inherent filtration is too high
2. tungsten target does not produce sufficient low energy photons
3. most diagnostic units are incapable of achieving appropriate focal-film distances

a. 1 and 2 only
b. 1 and 3 only
c. 2 and 3 only
d. 1, 2, & 3

129. What is the approximate average thickness of a fully compressed breast? **4**³⁰

135
D

a. 2 cm
b. 4 cm
c. 6 cm
d. 10 cm

130. What is the minimum number of ion chambers recommended for mammographic equipment in order to accommodate different breast sizes? **4**³¹

136
D

a. 2
b. 3
c. 4
d. 5

4³²   131.   What is the recommended kVp range for mammography?

       a.   7-10 kVp
       b.   17-20 kVp
       c.   20-35 kVp   B ¹²⁶
       d.   35-40 kVp

4³³   132.   What material is used to form the low energy absorbing window of a mammographic x-ray tube?

       a.   molybdenum
       b.   tungsten
       c.   beryllium
       d.   glass

1³⁴   133.   What is the required relationship between the emulsion surface of the film, the intensifying screen, and the patient?   A ¹²⁷

       1.   emulsion and screen toward patient
       2.   patient and emulsion toward screen
       3.   patient and screen away from emulsion

       a.   1 and 2 only
       b.   1 and 3 only
       c.   2 and 3 only
       d.   1, 2, & 3

134.   What is the recommended kVp level when screen-film contact tests are performed?   1³⁵

D ¹⁴⁰

a.   28 kVp
b.   38 kVp
c.   48 kVp
d.   58 kVp

135.   Which of the following are characteristics of single emulsion-single screen combinations?   1³⁶

1.   reduced speed
2.   increased detail
3.   decreased expense

B ¹⁴¹

a.   1 only
b.   2 only
c.   3 only
d.   1, 2, & 3

136.   Which of the following may produce poor film-screen contact?   2³⁴

C ¹⁴²

1.   dirt
2.   air
3.   cassette warping

a.   1 and 2 only
b.   1 and 3 only
c.   2 and 3 only
d.   1, 2, & 3

B ¹⁴³

2³⁵ 137. Which of the following is the primary benefit of using faster film-screen combinations?

a.   improved definition
b.   reduced graininess
c.   reduced patient dose   C¹³¹
d.   reduced latitude

2³⁶ 138. Which of the following affect image contrast?

1.   film characteristics
2.   processing conditions
3.   tissue absorption

a.   1 and 2 only   C¹³²
b.   1 and 3 only
c.   2 and 3 only
d.   1, 2, & 3

3³⁴ 139. Which of the following cassette sizes are recommended for mammography?

1.   24 x 35 cm
2.   24 x 30 cm
3.   18 x 24 cm

a.   1 and 2 only
b.   1 and 3 only
c.   2 and 3 only   A¹³³
d.   1, 2, & 3

140. Why are mammography cassettes constructed with thin sides? **3**³⁵

B ¹⁴⁷

   a. to decrease attenuation
   b. to increase film speed
   c. to increase film latitude
   d. to permit the film edge to demonstrate the chest wall

141. How is the emulsion side of a single emulsion film determined in the darkroom while loading a cassette? **3**³⁶

   a. it has a shinney surface
   b. it has a dull surface
   c. it appears a dull orange
   d. it appears a bright yellow

D ¹⁴⁸

142. What is the recommended storage temperature for radiographic film? **4**³⁴

   a. 20-40° F
   b. 40-50° F
   c. 60-70° F
   d. 80-90° F

143. What is the recommended humidity level for radiographic film storage? **4**³⁵

D ¹⁴⁹

   a. 10-20%
   b. 30-60%
   c. 70-80%
   d. 90-100%

4[36]   144.   Which layer of the intensifying screen is closest to the x-ray film emulsion?

a.   protective coating
b.   phosphor
c.   reflective   C [137]
d.   base

1[37]   145.   Which of the following are critical for sensitometric procedures?

1.   insert the less exposed end of the sensitometric strip into the processor first
2.   insert all sensitometric strips on the same side of the processor feed tray
3.   wait at least 2 hours between exposing and processing a sensitometric strip   D [138]

a.   1 and 2 only
b.   1 and 3 only
c.   2 and 3 only
d.   1, 2, & 3

1[38]   146.   What is the recommended optical density (OD) range for the speed step (speed index or mid density) when charting sensitometric results?   C [139]

a.   0.20
b.   0.50
c.   1.25
d.   2.50

147. How often is it recommended that the mammography darkroom be cleaned?

1^{39}

a. after each examination
b. daily

D^{153}

c. weekly
d. monthly

148. Which of the following are valid reasons for conducting a retake or reject analysis?

1^{40}

1. reduce cost
2. reduce patient exposures
3. evaluate the causes of repeated exposures

a. 1 and 2 only
b. 1 and 3 only
c. 2 and 3 only
d. 1, 2, & 3

C^{154}

149. What is the effect on the film image when insufficient replenishment occurs in a film processor due to a quantity of large size films being run with the replenishment set for an average size film?

1^{41}

a. density increases, contrast increases
b. density increases, contrast decreases
c. density decreases, contrast increases
d. density decreases, contrast decreases

1⁴²   150.   What term describes an undesirable marking on a mammogram that is produced from handling, storage, or processing?

     a.   blur
     b.   artifact   144
     c.   lag   A
     d.   line spread function

1⁴³   151.   What device is used to produce an optical sensitometric step wedge on a film?

     a.   densitometer
     b.   dosimeter
     c.   sensitometer
     d.   penetrometer

1⁴⁴   152.   Which of the following affect the quantity of safelight illumination in a darkroom?

     1.   type of filter
     2.   wattage of light source
     3.   distance of light from film loading   145
           surface   A

     a.   1 and 2 only
     b.   1 and 3 only
     c.   2 and 3 only
     d.   1, 2, & 3

146
C

Instrumentation

153. What classification of artifact would include pi lines?   **2**³⁷

    a.   exposure
    b.   handling

¹⁵⁸
B   c.   storage
    d.   processing

154. Why should mercury thermometers be avoided when measuring processor developer temperature?   **2**³⁸

    1.   mercury does not measure developer temperature accurately
    2.   mercury coagulates above 92° F
    3.   if broken mercury could permanently contaminate the developer tank

¹⁵⁹
A   a.   1 only
    b.   2 only
    c.   3 only
    d.   1, 2, & 3

¹⁶⁰
B

2^{39} 155. Which of the following is a potential problem when darkroom humidity is too high?

1. water condensation on films may produce water droplet artifacts
2. static artifacts are more easily produced
3. half moon artifacts are more likely

B ^{150}

a. 1 only
b. 2 only
c. 3 only
d. 1, 2, & 3

2^{40} 156. Which automatic film processing system is responsible for pressure artifacts?

C ^{151}

a. temperature control
b. transport
c. circulation
d. dryer

2^{41} 157. Which of the following should be recorded during a retake/reject analysis?

1. exposure factors
2. positioning
3. waste

D ^{152}

a. 1 and 2 only
b. 1 and 3 only
c. 2 and 3 only
d. 1, 2, & 3

Instrumentation

158. What is considered the average size of the compressed breast for an accreditation phantom?

    a.   2.5 cm
    b.   4.5 cm
    c.   6.5 cm
    d.   8.5 cm

2^{42}

159. What effect is produced by developer underreplenishment?

B[163]

    1.   decreased image density
    2.   decreased image contrast
    3.   fixer contamination

    a.   1 and 2 only
    b.   1 and 3 only
    c.   2 and 3 only
    d.   1, 2, & 3

2^{43}

B[164]   160. What is the minimum patient volume required for a meaningful mammographic film repeat/reject study according to the American College of Radiology?

    a.   100
    b.   250
A[165]   c.   500
    d.   1,000

2^{44}

3^{37} 161. If cleaning an intensifying screen does not remove small areas of poor contact, what should be the next step to solve the problem?

1. tighten the hinges
2. replace the screen
3. replace the foam behind the screen

a. 1 and 2 only
b. 1 and 3 only
c. 2 and 3 only
d. 1, 2, & 3

3^{38} 162. What is the maximum percentage difference permissible between the primary x-ray beam field and the collimator light field?

a. 0.5
b. 1.0
c. 1.5
d. 2.0

A ^{155}

B ^{156}

D ^{157}

163. If a non-dedicated film processing unit is used for mammographic films, which of the following become potential quality control problems?

3^{39}

1. volume fluxuations may cause the developer solution to become hyperactive or hypoactive
2. decreased image noise
3. decreased image contrast

a. 1 and 2 only
b. 1 and 3 only
c. 2 and 3 only
d. 1, 2, & 3

B ^{168}

164. How often should mammographic intensifying screens be cleaned?

3^{40}

a. after each examination
b. weekly
c. monthly
d. twice a year

D ^{169}

165. What causes a curtain effect artifact?

3^{41}

a. processing
b. exposure
c. film handling
d. film storage

C ^{170}

3⁴² 166. Which of the following should be checked regularly as part of a total mammographic quality control program?

1. darkroom fog level
2. viewboxes
3. compression device

a. 1 and 2 only
b. 1 and 3 only
c. 2 and 3 only   C ¹⁶¹
d. 1, 2, & 3

3⁴³ 167. Which of the following are valid justifications for the use of extended mammographic film processing?

1. increased contrast
2. reduced radiation dose
3. increased tube life   D ¹⁶²

a. 1 only
b. 2 only
c. 3 only
d. 1, 2, & 3

168. Which of the following is a potential problem when darkroom humidity is too low?

3⁴⁴

174
A

1. water condensation on films may produce water droplet artifacts
2. static artifacts are more easily produced
3. half moon artifacts are more likely

a. 1 only
b. 2 only
c. 3 only
d. 1, 2, & 3

169. What kVp setting is required for quality control exposures of an accreditation phantom?

4³⁷

175
D

a. 22
b. 24
c. 26
d. 28

170. Approximately how often should the fluorescent tubes in viewboxes be replaced?

4³⁸

176
B

a. every month
b. 3-4 months
c. 18-24 months
d. 60-72 months

┌ Simulated Exam   Question # ┐
┌ Question #   Answer ┐
↓ ↓   ↓ ↓

4^{39} 171.   What is the purpose of scoring or rating accreditation phantom images?

     a.   determination of accreditation status
     b.   comparative quality control
     c.   patient radiation dose calculation
     d.   evaluation of film-screen contact

4^{40} 172.   Which of the following is a recommended procedure for measuring developer temperature? D^{166}

     a.   measure directly in the developer tank
     b.   record measurements after each film
     c.   compare measurements to fixer temperature
     d.   chart measurements once a month

4^{41} 173.   What type of artifact is produced by small opaque foreign bodies collecting on an intensifying screen?

     a.   decreased density D^{167}
     b.   increased density
     c.   quantum mottle
     d.   branching densities

174.   What device is used to produce optical density measurements from an optical step wedge on a film?   **4**⁴²

   a.   densitometer
   b.   dosimeter
   c.   sensitometer
   d.   penetrometer

175.   Which of the following is a possible cause of film fog?   **4**⁴³

   1.   expired film date
   2.   improper safelight conditions
   3.   exposure of film to chemical fumes

   a.   1 only
   b.   2 only
   c.   3 only
   d.   1, 2, & 3

176.   What occurs to film sensitivity after exposure?   **4**⁴⁴

   a.   it decreases
   b.   it is increased 2X
   c.   it is increased 4X
   d.   it is increased 10X

B¹⁸¹

1⁴⁵   177.   Where is the skin covering the breast normally thickest?

    a.   base
    b.   areola
    c.   nipple
    d.   axillary prolongation (tail)

B¹⁷¹

1⁴⁶   178.   Which quadrant of the breast includes most of the glandular tissue?

    a.   lower outer
    b.   upper outer
    c.   lower inner
    d.   upper inner

1⁴⁷   179.   What term describes the fascial bands that support the breast?

A¹⁷²

    a.   Cooper's ligaments
    b.   parenchymal tissue
    c.   superficial fascia
    d.   pectoral muscle

2⁴⁵   180.   How many lobes are normally contained in each breast?

A¹⁷³

    a.   2-3
    b.   5-10
    c.   15-20
    d.   30-35

┌─ Answer
│ ┌─ Question #

                                    Question # ─┐
                          Simulated Exam ─┐ │
                                              │
↓ ↓   ↓ ↓

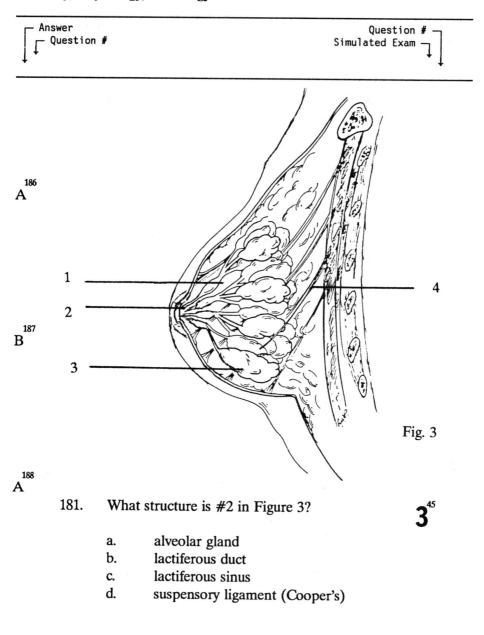

186
A

187
B

Fig. 3

188
A

181.   What structure is #2 in Figure 3?   **3**⁴⁵

a.   alveolar gland
b.   lactiferous duct
c.   lactiferous sinus
d.   suspensory ligament (Cooper's)

189
A

3⁴⁶ 182. What structure is #1 in Figure 3?

    a.   alveolar gland
    b.   lactiferous duct
    c.   lactiferous sinus   A¹⁷⁷
    d.   suspensory ligament (Cooper's)

3⁴⁷ 183. What structure is #4 in Figure 3?

    a.   alveolar gland
    b.   lactiferous duct
    c.   lactiferous sinus
    d.   suspensory ligament (Cooper's)

2⁴⁶ 184. What term describes the cone-shaped   B¹⁷⁸
structure that lies just beneath the areola?

    a.   ampulla
    b.   inframammary crease
    c.   retromammary space
    d.   tail of Spence

2⁴⁷ 185. Which of the following describes the junction   A¹⁷⁹
between the inferior part of the breast and
the anterior chest wall?

    a.   axillary tail
    b.   inframammary crease
    c.   retromammary space   ¹⁸⁰
    d.   tail of Spence   C

186.   Which of the following arteries supply the breast?   **2**⁴⁵

    a.   lateral thoracic
    b.   brachiocephalic
    c.   subclavian
    d.   superior vena cava

192
D

187.   Of what type of tissue is the nipple made?   **4**⁴⁶

    a.   fatty
    b.   erectile
    c.   fibroglandular
    d.   glandular

188.   Which muscle underlies the base of the breast?   **4**⁴⁷

    a.   pectoralis major
    b.   pectoralis minor
    c.   axillary tail
    d.   clavipectoral fascia

189.   Which of the following changes in the breast lobules accompany increasing age?   **1**⁴⁸

    1.   decreased size
    2.   decreased number
    3.   change to fibroglandular tissue

    a.   1 and 2 only
    b.   1 and 3 only
    c.   2 and 3 only
    d.   1, 2, & 3

Anatomy, Physiology, Pathology

┌─ Simulated Exam
│ ┌─ Question #
│ │   Question # ─┐
│ │   Answer ─┐ │
↓ ↓   ↓ ↓

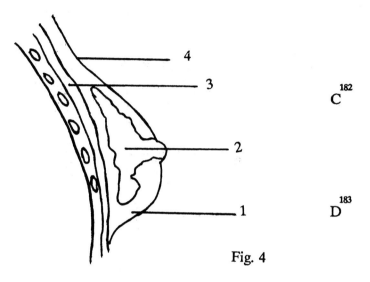

Fig. 4

182
C

183
D

1⁴⁹ 190. What structure is #2 in Figure 4?

    a.   skin
    b.   pectoralis major muscle
    c.   glandular tissue
    d.   adipose tissue

184
A

1⁵⁰ 191. What type of tissue comprises the stroma?

    1.   adipose
    2.   connective
    3.   glandular

185
B

    a.   1 and 2 only
    b.   1 and 3 only
    c.   2 and 3 only
    d.   1, 2, & 3

192.   Which of the following arteries supply the breast?

1⁵¹

1.   lateral thoracic branch of the axillary
2.   intercostal
3.   internal mammary branches

a.   1 and 2 only
b.   1 and 3 only
c.   2 and 3 only
d.   1, 2, & 3

197
C

198
C

199
B

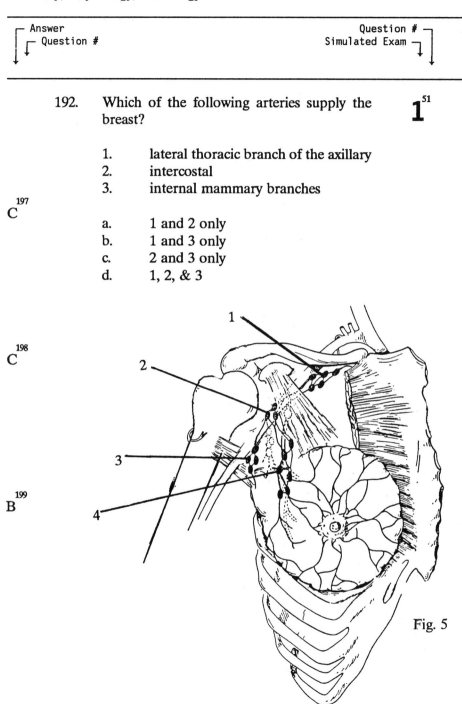

Fig. 5

2⁴⁸   193.   What lymphatic subgroup is represented by #4 in Figure 5?

     a.   pectoral
     b.   lateral
     c.   apical
     d.   central

2⁴⁹   194.   What lymphatic subgroup is represented by #1 in Figure 5?

     a.   pectoral
     b.   lateral
     c.   apical
     d.   central

2⁵⁰   195.   Which of the following is the milk producing unit of the breast?

     a.   acinus
     b.   sebaceous glands
     c.   Morgagni's tubercles   C ¹⁹⁰
     d.   Rotter's nodes

2⁵¹   196.   Which veins supply drainage for the breast?

     1.   axillary
     2.   intercostal
     3.   internal mammary

     a.   1 only
     b.   2 only
     c.   3 only   A ¹⁹¹
     d.   1, 2, & 3

197. Approximately how many axillary lymphatic nodes are there in a normal breast?   **3**⁴⁸

    a.   1-3
    b.   5-10
    c.   12-30
    d.   40-56

198. Which intercostal nerve is the primary sensory nerve to the nipple-areolar complex?   **3**⁴⁹

    a.   2nd
    b.   3rd
    c.   4th
    d.   5th

199. What term describes the area between the posterior aspect of the glandular tissue and the anterior aspect of the pectoral muscle?   **3**⁵⁰

    a.   axillary tail
    b.   retromammary space
    c.   inframammary crease
    d.   papillary channels

C²⁰³

3[51]   200.   Which of the following is correct regarding the location of the pectoralis minor muscle in relation to the pectoralis major?

   1.   posterior
   2.   inferior   A[193]
   3.   medial

   a.   1 only
   b.   2 only
   c.   3 only
   d.   1, 2, & 3

4[48]   201.   What tissue primarily constitutes the postpubertal adolescent breast?   C[194]

   a.   connective
   b.   adipose
   c.   glandular
   d.   subcutaneous

4[49]   202.   Which of the following is true regarding the retromammary space?   A[195]

   1.   it lies anterior to the pectoral major muscle
   2.   it lies anterior to the glandular tissue
   3.   contains mostly adipose tissue

   a.   1 and 2 only
   b.   1 and 3 only
   c.   2 and 3 only   D[196]
   d.   1, 2, & 3

83

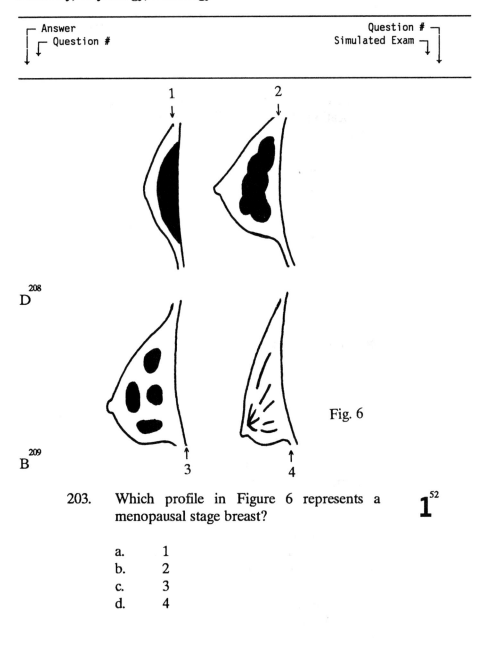

Fig. 6

208
D

209
B

203. Which profile in Figure 6 represents a menopausal stage breast?

1[52]

a.   1
b.   2
c.   3
d.   4

210
D

2^{52} 204. Which profile in Figure 6 represents a senescent stage breast?

    a.   1
    b.   2
    c.   3
    d.   4

2^{53} 205. Which profile in Figure 6 represents a pre-pregnancy stage breast?

                                                   200
                                               A

    a.   1
    b.   2
    c.   3
    d.   4

4^{50} 206. Which of the following is a milk-like fluid that is secreted during pregnancy from the breasts?

                                                   201
                                               A

    a.   melanoblast
    b.   colostrum
    c.   carotene
    d.   synovium

4^{51} 207. Which group of lymph nodes receive most of the lymph from the upper limb and drain into the central node group?

    a.   apical
    b.   lateral
    c.   subscapular   202
    d.   pectoral   B

208. Which of the following are types of breast tissue?

    1 ^{53}

    1. fibrous
    2. glandular
    3. adipose

    a. 1 and 2 only
    b. 1 and 3 only
    c. 2 and 3 only
    d. 1, 2, & 3

209. Which of the following are true regarding breast tissues?

    1 ^{54}

^{214}
D

    1. adipose tissue is less dense
    2. glandular tissue is less dense
    3. connective tissue is more dense

    a. 1 and 2 only
    b. 1 and 3 only
    c. 2 and 3 only
    d. 1, 2, & 3

^{215}
A

210. Which of the following affect the relative density of the breast tissue?

    2 ^{54}

    1. age
    2. number of pregnancies
    3. hormone status

    a. 1 and 2 only
    b. 1 and 3 only
    c. 2 and 3 only
    d. 1, 2, & 3

3^{52} 211. Which of the following describes the embryologic origin of the female breasts?

    a.   sebaceous gland
    b.   hair follicle
    c.   aprocrine sweat gland
    d.   skin pore D^{204}

3^{53} 212. Which of the following categories of breasts are primarily fatty tissue?

    1.   male
    2.   female over 50
    3.   female lactating

                                                A^{205}

    a.   1 and 2 only
    b.   1 and 3 only
    c.   2 and 3 only
    d.   1, 2, & 3

3^{54} 213. Which of the following patients would be expected to exhibit fibro-glandular breasts?

                                                B^{206}

    1.   childless females over age 30
    2.   females between age 15 and 30
    3.   males

    a.   1 and 2 only
    b.   1 and 3 only
    c.   2 and 3 only
    d.   1, 2, & 3

                                                B^{207}

214.   Which of the following describe the 4^{52}
        distribution of fibrous connective tissue and
        ducts?

        1.   they are irregularly superimposed
              throughout the breast
        2.   the trabeculae arise from the broad
              base of the chest wall
        3.   they are located between the
              superficial and deep layers of
              superficial fascia

        a.   1 and 2 only
C ^{219} b.   1 and 3 only
        c.   2 and 3 only
        d.   1, 2, & 3

215.   Which of the following best describes the 4^{53}
        effect of childbearing and advancing age on
        the glandular tissue of the breast?

        a.   atrophy
        b.   introsusception
        c.   lactation
        d.   crystallization

B ^{220}

4^{54} 216. Which of the following patients would be expected to exhibit fibro-fatty breasts?

1. males
2. females between age 15 and 30
3. middle aged females with 3 or more pregnancies

211
C

a. 1 only
b. 2 only
c. 3 only
d. 1, 2, & 3

1^{55} 217. What term describes the progressive degeneration that occurs naturally with advancing age, resulting in a shriveling of the organs or tissues?

212
A

a. involution
b. inversion
c. intromission
d. intervertigo

1^{56} 218. Which of the following hormones play an important role in breast development and lactation?

1. insulin
2. growth hormone
3. corticosteroids

213
A

a. 1 and 2 only
b. 1 and 3 only
c. 2 and 3 only
d. 1, 2, & 3

219. Which of the following may assist women in tolerating compression by decreasing breast sensitivity?

1^{57}

1. avoid using deodorants immediately prior to mammography
2. decrease caffeine 2 weeks prior to mammography
3. perform mammography during the week after menses

²²⁴
C

a. 1 and 2 only
b. 1 and 3 only
c. 2 and 3 only
d. 1, 2, & 3

220. Which of the following are normal as a result of the onset of menstruation?

2^{55}

²²⁵
D

1. regression of the lobules
2. replacement of parenchymal tissue by fat
3. involution of the terminal ductal lobular unit

a. 1 and 2 only
b. 1 and 3 only
c. 2 and 3 only
d. 1, 2, & 3

²²⁶
A

2⁵⁶ 221. Approximately how long does the process of atrophy of mammary structures that commences at menopause last?

    a.   1 year
    b.   3-5 years
    c.   8-10 years
    d.   15-20 years

2⁵⁷ 222. Which of the following is caused by estrogen? C²¹⁶

    a.   lobular proliferation and growth
    b.   ductal proliferation
    c.   increase in fatty tissue
    d.   involution of the senescent breast

3⁵⁵ 223. What type of tissue replaces supportive tissue during involution?

    a.   glandular A²¹⁷
    b.   connective
    c.   fatty
    d.   fibrous

D²¹⁸

224. Why is nursing the baby desirable when mammography must be performed on the lactating breast?

3^{56}

C^{230}

    a. nursing stimulates estrogen production which will enhance benign masses

    b. involution of the lobules and ducts will begin when nursing ends

    c. removal of superimposed milk increases tissue visualization

    d. removal of milk reduces milk-based artifacts

225. What is the final region of the breast to undergo menopausal involution?

3^{57}

D^{231}

    a. lateral
    b. medial
    c. posterior
    d. nipple

226. Which of the following are normal results of involution?

4^{55}

A^{232}

    1. pendulous breasts
    2. benign fatty lumps
    3. lobular proliferation

    a. 1 and 2 only
    b. 1 and 3 only
    c. 2 and 3 only
    d. 1, 2, & 3

4⁵⁶   227.   Which portions of the breast begin to atrophy first at menopause?

    1.   medial
    2.   lateral
    3.   posterior

²²¹
B

    a.   1 and 2 only
    b.   1 and 3 only
    c.   2 and 3 only
    d.   1, 2, & 3

4⁵⁷   228.   Which of the following is caused by progesterone?

²²²
B

    a.   lobular proliferation and growth
    b.   ductal proliferation
    c.   increase in fatty tissue
    d.   involution of the senescent breast

1⁵⁸   229.   Which of the following are benign diseases of the breast?

²²³
C

    1.   adenosis
    2.   apocrine metaplasia (apocrine change)
    3.   sebaceous cyst

    a.   1 and 2 only
    b.   1 and 3 only
    c.   2 and 3 only
    d.   1, 2, & 3

230. What is the most common benign breast neoplasm? **1**⁵⁹

    a.   lymphangiosarcoma
    b.   lobular adenocarcinoma
    c.   fibroadenoma
    d.   florid adenoma of the nipple

C²³⁶

231. Which of the following aspects of nipple discharges have clinical significance? **1**⁶⁰

    1.   persistent
    2.   nonlactational
    3.   unilateral

    a.   1 and 2 only
    b.   1 and 3 only
    c.   2 and 3 only
    d.   1, 2, & 3

D²³⁷

232. Which of the following is a primary presentation of mammographic pathology? **1**⁶¹

    a.   mass
    b.   unilateral pain
    c.   bilateral nodularity
    d.   asymmetry

B²³⁸

1⁶² 233. What is architectural distortion?

    a. radial lines converging at the nipple
    b. diametric lines converging at the nipple
    c. interruption of the natural flow towards the nipple
    d. patterns resulting from surgical intervention

2⁵⁸ 234. Which of the following is the most common type of breast carcinoma?   B²²⁷

    a. ductal adenocarcinoma
    b. medullary carcinoma
    c. mucinous carcinoma
    d. tubular carcinoma

2⁵⁹ 235. Which of the following is a common presentation of a lipoma?   A²²⁸

    1. radiolucent
    2. encapsulated
    3. easily moveable

    a. 1 only
    b. 2 only
    c. 3 only
    d. 1, 2, & 3

D²²⁹

236. Approximately what percentage of calcifications represent malignant breast disease?   **2**^{60}

  a. 5-10
  b. 20-30
  c. 40-50
  d. 70-80

237. Which of the following are potential causes of edema of the breast?   **2**^{61}

242
A

  1. carcinoma
  2. obstruction of the lymphatics
  3. inflammatory disease

  a. 1 and 2 only
  b. 1 and 3 only
  c. 2 and 3 only
  d. 1, 2, & 3

238. Which of the following mammographic characteristics of calcifications are usually indications of malignant disease?   **2**^{62}

243
A

  1. varying densities
  2. well defined borders
  3. unilateral

  a. 1 and 2 only
  b. 1 and 3 only
  c. 2 and 3 only
  d. 1, 2, & 3

3^{58} 239.   Which of the following mammographic characteristics of calcifications are usually indications of benign disease?

1.   arterial
2.   popcorn type
3.   rim

233
C

a.   1 and 2 only
b.   1 and 3 only
c.   2 and 3 only
d.   1, 2, & 3

3^{59} 240.   Which of the following are considered to be secondary features of breast malignancy?

234
A

1.   skin thickening and/or retraction
2.   axillary lymph node enlargement
3.   more than two discreet masses

a.   1 and 2 only
b.   1 and 3 only
c.   2 and 3 only
d.   1, 2, & 3

3^{60} 241.   Which of the following is often the only early sign of malignancy?

235
D

a.   micro-calcifications
b.   masses
c.   nipple retraction
d.   skin thickening

242.   Which of the following would be expected of an infiltrating carcinoma of the breast?   **3**⁶¹

D²⁴⁷

1.   extremely hard on palpation
2.   larger on palpation than the mammographic image
3.   oval configuration and smooth margin

a.   1 and 2 only
b.   1 and 3 only
c.   2 and 3 only
d.   1, 2, & 3

243.   Which of the following are considered the primary signs of mammographic masses that are malignant?   **3**⁶²

D²⁴⁸

1.   dense
2.   irregular margins
3.   follow normal architecture

a.   1 and 2 only
b.   1 and 3 only
c.   2 and 3 only
d.   1, 2, & 3

4⁵⁸   244.   Which of the following are aspects of calcifications that usually require biopsy?

1.   new
2.   increased number
3.   decreased density

a.   1 and 2 only
b.   1 and 3 only
c.   2 and 3 only
d.   1, 2, & 3

D ²³⁹

4⁵⁹   245.   Which of the following are common causes of breast calcifications?

1.   thickened and dried secretions
2.   necrosis
3.   atrophy

a.   1 and 2 only
b.   1 and 3 only
c.   2 and 3 only
d.   1, 2, & 3

A ²⁴⁰

4⁶⁰   246.   Which of the following is a primary presentation of mammographic pathology?

a.   edema
b.   increased connective tissue density
c.   masses
d.   nipple discharge

A ²⁴¹

247. When are breast cysts most common?

4^{61}

a. during pregnancy
b. during lactation
c. adolescent
d. menopausal

C [252]

248. Which of the following should be considered in determining whether calcifications should be biopsied?

4^{62}

1. distribution
2. surrounding tissue or associated mass
3. density

a. 1 and 2 only
b. 1 and 3 only
C [253]
c. 2 and 3 only
d. 1, 2, & 3

B [254]

1⁶³ 249. What portion of the breast is best demonstrated by the CC position?

    a. axillary
    b. inframammary crease
    c. subareolar
    d. tail

1⁶⁴ 250. Which area of the breast is visualized on the CC position but not on the MLO?

A²⁴⁴

    1. axillary
    2. medial
    3. subareolar

    a. 1 only
    b. 2 only
    c. 3 only
    d. 1, 2, & 3

1⁶⁵ 251. Where should the opposite arm be placed when positioning for the CC position?

A²⁴⁵

    a. forward (holding onto a handle bar when available)
    b. relaxed at the side
    c. relaxed in external rotation at the side
    d. flexed at the elbow, with hand on hip

C²⁴⁶

252. Where should the arm on the side of the body being imaged be placed when positioning for the CC position?

1^{66}

a. forward (holding onto a handle bar when available)
b. tensed and at the side
c. relaxed in external rotation at the side
d. flexed at the elbow, with hand on hip

B^{258} 253. What is the proper angle between the inframammary crease and the chest wall to determine the proper height of the image receptor for the CC position?

1^{67}

a. 10°
b. 45°
c. 90°
d. 180°

D^{259} 254. Which area/s of the breast is/are not imaged on the CC position?

1^{68}

1. inferior anterior
2. superior posterior
3. medial central

a. 1 only
b. 2 only
c. 3 only
d. 1, 2, & 3

B^{260}

1[69] 255. What is the proper position for the patient's head during the CC position of the right breast?

    a.   straight ahead
    b.   neck extended
    c.   turned to the right
    d.   turned to the left

C [249]

1[70] 256. Which of the following areas is not visualized on the CC position?

    a.   axillary
    b.   central
    c.   medial
    d.   subareolar

2[63] 257. Which of the following is the proper action if the breast is positioned correctly for the CC position, but the nipple is not in profile?

B [250]

    a.   adjust the technical factors for a lower density
    b.   reposition the breast until the nipple is in profile
    c.   perform an additional position for the anterior breast only with the nipple in profile
    d.   attempt a caudal-cephalic position

A [251]

    Question #

                                                            Question #
                                                        Simulated Exam

258.   Which of the following is recommended to
        remove wrinkling of the skin surface in the
        axillary area when positioning for a CC
        position?

2^{64}

    a.   oblique the patient 45° to the
         opposite side

    b.   place the arm of the affected side in
         a different position

    c.   reduce compression

    d.   move the patient back from the
         image receptor tray

264
A

259.   Which of the following will insure the
        inclusion of all medial tissue during the CC
        position?

2^{65}

    a.   perform a caudal-cephalo position

    b.   rotate the tube (or C-arm) 10°

    c.   turn the head toward the affected side

    d.   place the opposite breast on the
         image receptor

265
A

260.   Which of the following are considered the
        routine positions for screening
        mammography?

2^{66}

    1.   CC
    2.   LMO
    3.   MLO

    a.   1 and 2 only
    b.   1 and 3 only
    c.   2 and 3 only
    d.   1, 2, & 3

2⁶⁷ 261. Which of the following is a recommended solution to performing the CC position on a kyphotic patient?

a. perform a caudo-cephalad position
b. raise both arms and place the hands behind the neck
c. rotate the tube (or C-arm) 15°
d. oblique the patient 30° toward the affected side

255
D

2⁶⁸ 262. What position of the arm will usually remove the fat fold in the axillary area for a CC position?

a. externally rotate the shoulder
b. internally rotate the shoulder
c. flex the elbow and place the hand on the hip
d. move the arm anteriorly

256
A

2⁶⁹ 263. Which of the following is recommended for the patient when performing the CC position?

a. place both arms on the head
b. lean back from the image receptor tray
c. stand 1/2 step back and lean in toward the image receptor tray
d. oblique the body 45°

257
C

264. Which of the following is true about the pectoral muscle on the CC position?

2^{70}

1. it is visualized occasionally
2. the use of curved paddles are required to visualize it satisfactorily
3. it is usually visualized in older patients only

B^{269}

a. 1 only
b. 2 only
c. 3 only
d. 1, 2, & 3

A^{270} 265. Which area of the breast is not visualized on the MLO position?

3^{63}

a. posterior medial
b. anterior medial
c. posterior lateral
d. anterior lateral

D^{271}

3⁶⁴ 266. The purpose of the MLO position is to:

1. along with the CC position, provide the primary screening mammography position
2. visualize as much of the axillary tail as possible
3. with the CC position, permit visualization of lesions in two planes

A²⁶¹

a. 1 and 2 only
b. 1 and 3 only
c. 2 and 3 only
d. 1, 2, & 3

3⁶⁵ 267. What plane is referred to when discussing obliques of the breast for the MLO position?

a. axis of the plane of compression
b. angle of the chest wall
c. angle between the inframammary crease and the chest wall
d. mid-sagittal line of the body

A²⁶²

3⁶⁶ 268. Which position demonstrates more tissue than the others?

a. MLO
b. CC
c. 90° LM
d. 90° ML

C²⁶³

269. What is the proper position of the x-ray tube C-arm when positioning for a MLO position?

3^{67}

a. perpendicular to the pectoral muscle
b. parallel to the pectoral muscle
c. parallel to the inframammary crease
d. perpendicular to the chest wall

B²⁷⁵

270. Which quadrant is best visualized with a MLO position?

3^{68}

a. upper outer
b. upper inner
c. lower outer
d. lower inner

D²⁷⁶

271. What is the approximate recommended tube angle for a MLO position of an asthenic patient?

3^{69}

a. 30°
b. 40°
c. 50°
d. 60°

B²⁷⁷

3⁷⁰ 272. Which of the following must be demonstrated on the MLO position?

1. pectoral muscle to the nipple
2. medial breast
3. inframammary crease

a. 1 and 2 only
b. 1 and 3 only
c. 2 and 3 only
d. 1, 2, & 3

4⁶³ 273. In what direction should the patient rotate the shoulder immediately prior to final compression for the MLO position to demonstrate as much of the pectoralis muscle as possible?

D²⁶⁶

a. anterior
b. posterior
c. inferior
d. superior

267
A

4⁶⁴ 274. Which of the following describes pectoralis excavatum, which presents problems in positioning the breast for a MLO position?

a. concave chest wall
b. depressed sternum
c. barrel chest
d. short torso

268
A

275.   In what direction should the breast tissue and
        pectoralis muscle be moved when positioning
        the breast for a MLO position?

        a.   anterior and medial
        b.   anterior and lateral

281   c.   posterior and medial
C   d.   posterior and lateral

276.   A line between what two anatomical
        landmarks will best determine the correct
        tube angle for a MLO position?

        a.   axilla and xiphoid
        b.   sternal notch and nipple
        c.   angle of 3rd rib to inframammary
              crease
        d.   shoulder to mid-sternum

277.   Why should a small quantity of tissue below
        the inframammary crease be demonstrated on
        a MLO position?

282
A
        1.   breast tissue sometimes extends into
              the rib interspaces
        2.   it insures that the breast has been
              demonstrated to the chest wall
        3.   major lymph nodes are located in
              this area

283
C   a.   1 only
        b.   2 only
        c.   3 only
        d.   1, 2, & 3

4^{65}

4^{66}

4^{67}

┌─ Simulated Exam   Question # ┐
│ ┌─ Question #   Answer   ┐ │
↓ ↓   ↓ ↓

4[68]   278.   The MLO position is preferred over the true lateral because of its effectiveness in visualizing which of the following?

1.   posterior breast
2.   upper outer quadrant
3.   upper inner quadrant

a.   1 and 2 only
b.   1 and 3 only
c.   2 and 3 only
d.   1, 2, & 3

B [272]

4[69]   279.   Where should the arm of the affected side be placed for a MLO position?

a.   relaxed and internally rotated
b.   flexed at the elbow with hand on hip
c.   forward to grasp the handlebar
d.   anteriorly with the hand internally rotated

A [273]

4[70]   280.   What is the range of tube angles used for the MLO position?

a.   0-30°
b.   40-70°
c.   80-90°
d.   100-130°

B [274]

Positioning

281. Which of the following positions would best demonstrate an extreme medial lesion of the breast? **1**⁷¹

    a.   axillary
    b.   exaggerated CC lateral
    c.   cleavage (valley view or double breast compressions)
    d.   MLO

C²⁸⁶

282. Which of the following are the primary reasons for performing a ML or LM 90° position of the breast? **1**⁷²

    1.   identification of the exact location of a lesion in the sagittal plane
    2.   demonstration of UIQ or LIQ tissue
    3.   demonstration of a maximum quantity of medial tissue

    a.   1 and 2 only
    b.   1 and 3 only
    c.   2 and 3 only
    d.   1, 2, & 3

283. Which position best demonstrates the effect of gravity or air-fluid/fat levels in the breast? **1**⁷³

    a.   CC
C²⁸⁷   b.   MLO
    c.   LM or ML
    d.   axillary tail

┌─ Simulated Exam   Question # ─┐
│ ┌─ Question #   Answer ┐ │
↓ ↓   ↓   ↓

1[74]   284.   Which of the following positions or techniques can be substituted for the MLO position for patients with pectoralis excavatum?

        a.   cleavage (valley view or double breast compressions)
        b.   coat hanger
        c.   LM or ML 90°
        d.   oblique lateral (Cleopatra)

[278]
A

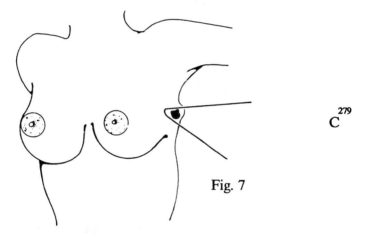

Fig. 7

[279]
C

1[75]   285.   Which of the following positions or techniques is being demonstrated in Figure 7?   [280] B

        a.   CC
        b.   coat hanger
        c.   exaggerated CC lateral
        d.   true lateral

Answer
Question #

Question #
Simulated Exam

286. In which portion of the breast is a lesion located if it appears higher on a 90° lateral position as compared to the MLO position? 1[76]

a. anterior

C[291] b. posterior

c. medial

d. lateral

C[292]

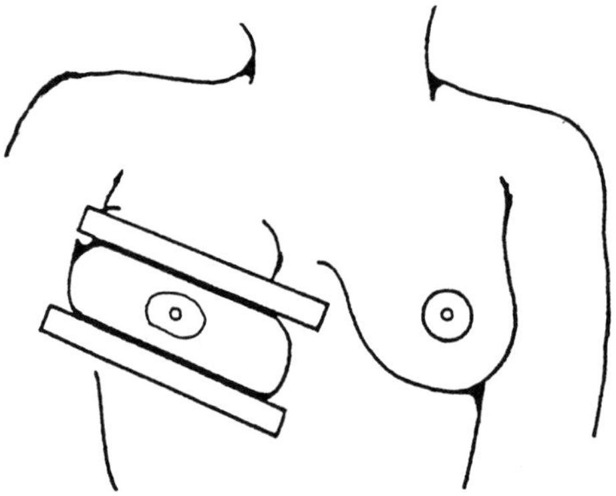

Fig. 8

287. Which of the following positions is being demonstrated in Figure 8? 1[77]

A[293]

a. axillary

b. mediolateral

c. 30° oblique

d. tangential

C[294]

2⁷¹   288.   What position is used to demonstrate tissue in the outer aspect of the breast that is not visualized on the routine CC position?

a.   tangential
b.   exaggerated CC lateral
c.   cleavage (valley view or double breast compressions)
d.   roll (turn view)

284
C

2⁷²   289.   Which of the following positions are recommended for post-operative open heart surgery patients or patients with a prominent pacemaker?

a.   MLO
b.   LMO
c.   true lateral
d.   exaggerated CC lateral

2⁷³   290.   Which angle would produce the best image of a right breast 1:00 lesion with a reverse LMO position?

a.   20°
b.   30°
c.   50°
d.   70°

285
B

Positioning

291. Which of the following positions or techniques is used to demonstrate tissue that has been superimposed on another position? 2^{74}

   a. axillary
   b. coat hanger
   c. roll (turn view)
   d. tangential

C^{296} 292. Which of the following positions is/are most helpful in demonstrating tissue in the 12:00 or 6:00 position? 2^{75}

   a. cleavage (valley view)
   b. exaggerated CC lateral
   c. ML 90° or LM 90°
   d. oblique lateral (Cleopatra)

C^{297} 293. Which position best demonstrates tissue that extends just beyond the lateral edge of the image receptor plate following the curve of the rib cage on the CC position? 2^{76}

   a. exaggerated CC lateral
   b. 30° oblique
   c. oblique lateral (Cleopatra)
   d. tangential

294. Which position best demonstrates deep axillary tissue? 2^{77}

B^{298}
   a. exaggerated CC lateral
   b. roll (turn view)
   c. oblique lateral (Cleopatra)
   d. tangential

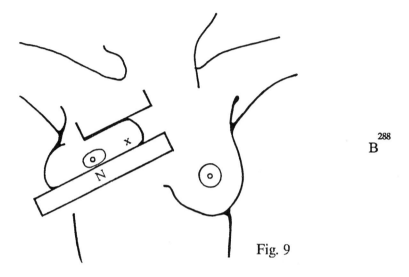

Fig. 9

B ^{288}

3^{71} 295.   Which of the following lesions will best be
demonstrated with the oblique projection in
Figure 9?

B ^{289}

     a.   12:00
     b.   2:30
     c.   5:30
     d.   8:30

D ^{290}

296.   Which additional position/s should be performed to determine if a lesion is milk of calcium?

3^{72}

1.   tangential
2.   roll (turn view)

302
C

3.   ML 90° or LM 90°

a.   1 only
b.   2 only
c.   3 only
d.   1, 2, & 3

297.   What position will project a questionable area in the breast as close as possible to the subcutaneous fat?

3^{73}

a.   CC
b.   MLO

303
B

c.   tangential
d.   ML 90° or LM 90°

298.   Which position/s is/are used to triangulate lesions?

3^{74}

1.   CC
2.   roll (turn view)
3.   MLO

304
A

a.   1 only
b.   2 only
c.   3 only
d.   1, 2, & 3

3[75]   299.   Which of the following positions are designed to assist in enhancing UOQ lesions?

1.   30° oblique
2.   exaggerated CC lateral
3.   oblique lateral (Cleopatra)

a.   1 and 2 only
b.   1 and 3 only
c.   2 and 3 only
d.   1, 2, & 3

3[76]   300.   Which angle would produce the best image of a right breast 2:30 lesion with a reverse LMO position?

a.   20°
b.   30°
c.   50°
d.   70°

3[77]   301.   Which position best demonstrates in a tangential position lesions in the superior or inferior breast regions best?

B[295]

a.   CC
b.   MLO
c.   LMO
d.   ML 90° or LM 90°

Positioning

302. Which position best demonstrates tissue that extends over the sternum?

4^{71}

a. CC
b. exaggerated CC lateral
c. cleavage (valley view or double breast compressions)
d. roll (turn view)

308
A

303. In which direction should breast tissue be pulled when positioning for a mediolateral lateral position?

4^{72}

1. superior
2. medial
3. lateral

a. 1 and 2 only
b. 1 and 3 only
c. 2 and 3 only
d. 1, 2, & 3

309
A

304. What is the primary objective of performing a 30° oblique position?

4^{73}

a. demonstrate the axillary tail and deep OUQ of the breast
b. demonstrate the inframammary crease
c. demonstrate medial tissue
d. demonstrate UIQ or LOQ tissue

310
A

4[74]   305.   Which of the following are indications for the coat hanger technique?

1.   a lesion outside compressible breast tissue
2.   a lesion very high on the chest wall
3.   a lesion very close to a silicone implant

a.   1 and 2 only
b.   1 and 3 only
c.   2 and 3 only
d.   1, 2, & 3

D [299]

4[75]   306.   What is the proper angulation for the oblique lateral (Cleopatra) when the patient does not straighten up?

a.   0°
b.   10°
c.   30°
d.   90°

A [300]

4[76]   307.   Which position best demonstrates a tangential view of lesions in the medial or lateral breast regions?

a.   CC
b.   MLO
c.   LMO
d.   ML 90° or LM 90°

D [301]

308. Which angle would produce the best image of a left breast 9:30 lesion with a reverse LMO position?   **4**[77]

    a.   20°
    b.   30°
    c.   50°
    d.   70°

A [314]

309. In what direction should the breast tissue be displaced when imaging the augmented breast with Eklund positioning?   **1**[78]

    1.   anteriorly
    2.   inferiorly
    3.   laterally

    a.   1 only
    b.   2 only
    c.   3 only
    d.   1, 2, & 3

C [315]

310. What position or technique is recommended for screening of post mastectomy patients?   **1**[79]

    a.   axillary
    b.   tangential
    c.   coat hanger
    d.   CC

1[80] 311. Which of the following is a potential solution to the problem created by extremely small breasts that will not remain under compression?

a. coat hanger technique
b. spot compression paddle
c. exaggerated CC lateral
d. cleavage (valley view or double breast compressions)

1[81] 312. Which of the following is/are recommended when the Eklund positions cannot be used to visualize the augmented breast?

D [305]

1. exaggerated CC lateral
2. cleavage (valley view or double breast compressions)
3. 90° lateral

A [306]

a. 1 only
b. 2 only
c. 3 only
d. 1, 2, & 3

2[78] 313. What position or technique best demonstrates recurring lesions along the chest wall of post mastectomy patients?

A [307]

a. axillary
b. tangential
c. coat hanger
d. CC

123

Positioning

314. Which of the following positions are recommended for a complete study of the augmented breast?

2[79]

1. routine CC and MLO
2. modified Eklund CC and MLO
3. 30° oblique

a. 1 and 2 only
b. 1 and 3 only
c. 2 and 3 only
d. 1, 2, & 3

315. Which of the following positions are required for a complete mammographic study of the unilateral post mastectomy breast?

2[80]

1. CC and MLO of affected breast
2. CC and MLO of unaffected breast
3. axillary of affected breast

B [318]

a. 1 and 2 only
b. 1 and 3 only
c. 2 and 3 only
d. 1, 2, & 3

2⁸¹ 316. Which of the following are contraindications for performing Eklund positions of the augmented breast?

1. tissue is firmly encapsulated and cannot be displaced posteriorly
2. little tissue is surrounding the implant
3. post mastectomy implants surrounded by skin only

311
B

a. 1 and 2 only
b. 1 and 3 only
c. 2 and 3 only
d. 1, 2, & 3

3⁷⁸ 317. Which of the following positions demonstrates the posterior tissue of the augmented breast?

1. CC
2. MLO
3. tangential

312
C

a. 1 and 2 only
b. 1 and 3 only
c. 2 and 3 only
d. 1, 2, & 3

313
A

Positioning

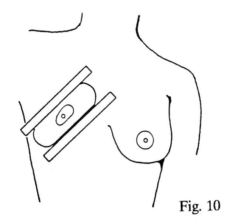

Fig. 10

321
C

318.   Which of the following positions is being demonstrated in Figure 10?

3^{79}

a.   cleavage
b.   lateromedial oblique
322
C   c.   exaggerated CC oblique
d.   roll (turn view)

323
A

126

3^{80} 319. Which of the following are rationale for utilizing Eklund positions for mammography of the augmented breast?

1. 2-5 cm of additional compression can be achieved
2. image detailed is enhanced by improved compression
3. significantly more tissue is visualized

a. 1 and 2 only
b. 1 and 3 only
c. 2 and 3 only
d. 1, 2, & 3

316
D

3^{81} 320. Which of the following positions or techniques can be performed on post mastectomy patients without compression while maintaining satisfactory quality of the mammogram?

a. axillary
b. tangential
c. coat hanger
d. CC

317
A

321. Which of the following will tighten the pectoral muscle, thus adding difficulty to positioning and compression? 4^{78}

   325
B

   1. slumping forward into poor posture
   2. raising the shoulder
   3. gripping the hand rail tightly

   a. 1 only
   b. 2 only
   c. 3 only
   d. 1, 2, & 3

322. Lesions at which location within the breast will best be visualized with a true lateral position? 4^{79}

   326
B

   a. 3:00 left or 9:00 right
   b. 3:00 right or 9:00 left
   c. 6:00 or 12:00
   d. 2:00 or 8:00

323. What position or technique should be performed to demonstrate recurrences of carcinoma on the affected side of post mastectomy patients? 4^{80}

   a. axillary
   b. tangential
   c. coat hanger

   327
B

   d. CC

4[81]   324.   In what direction should the prosthesis be displaced when positioning the augmented breast with Eklund positions?

1. posteriorly
2. inferiorly
3. superiorly

a. 1 and 2 only
b. 1 and 3 only
c. 2 and 3 only
d. 1, 2, & 3

D [319]

A [320]

325. Toward what structure does breast tissue move when compression is applied properly?   **1**^{82}

a. chest wall
b. nipple
c. axilla
d. clavicle

326. What is the primary goal of compression?   **1**^{83}

a. reduce patient motion
b. uniformly reduce the thickness of the breast

331
C

c. permit the use of an automatic exposure control (phototimer)
d. reduce image contrast

327. Which of the following are true regarding the use of motorized foot control compression?   **1**^{84}

1. it leaves both hands free to position the breast
2. it is most useful during the final stages of compression
3. it is most often used only during the first stage of compression

332
B

a. 1 and 2 only
b. 1 and 3 only
c. 2 and 3 only
d. 1, 2, & 3

2^{82} 328. Which of the following is true regarding good breast compression?

   1. it reduces object to film distance
   2. it separates internal structures for better visualization
   3. it reduces scatter radiation

   a. 1 and 2 only
   b. 1 and 3 only
   c. 2 and 3 only
   d. 1, 2, & 3

   B^{324}

2^{83} 329. What is the guideline for adequate compression?

   a. the nipple begins to invert
   b. breast tissue can be easily indented by the fingertips
   c. breast tissue is firm and taut to the touch
   d. the patient objects

2^{84} 330. Which of the following produces a more homogenous film density as a result of vigorous compression?

   a. posterior and anterior tissue is spread to an even thickness
   b. glandular tissue is moved toward the chest wall
   c. the pectoral muscle is pulled away from the chest wall
   d. scatter radiation is increased

331.   Which of the following are reasons why vigorous compression permits more accurate evaluation of masses?

3⁸²

1.   carcinomas are more easily compressed than benign tumors
2.   cysts are more easily compressed than carcinomas
3.   normal glandular tissue is more easily compressed than carcinomas

a.   1 and 2 only
b.   1 and 3 only
c.   2 and 3 only
d.   1, 2, & 3

³³⁵
A

332.   What effect does vigorous compression have on image quality as compared to poor compression of the same breast?

3⁸³

1.   increases contrast
2.   decreases density
3.   increased detail

a.   1 and 2 only
b.   1 and 3 only
c.   2 and 3 only
d.   1, 2, & 3

³³⁶
C

132

3⁸⁴ 333. Which of the following describes the development of new lobular units or their enlargement?

1. sebaceous cyst
2. gynecomastia
3. adenosis

a. 1 only
b. 2 only
c. 3 only
d. 1, 2, & 3

D ³²⁸

4⁸² 334. Which of the following compression devices are acceptable for use with film-screen mammography?

1. spot
2. curved
3. flat 90° to the plane of the chest wall

a. 1 and 2 only
b. 1 and 3 only
c. 2 and 3 only
d. 1, 2, & 3

C ³²⁹

A ³³⁰

335.   What is recommended when compression causes the nipple not to appear in profile?

4^{83}

    a.   avoid repositioning and sacrificing the demonstration of tissue in another direction

    b.   perform an additional axillary tail position to demonstrate the nipple in profile

340
A

    c.   pull breast tissue from the inframammary crease to permit the nipple to go into profile

    d.   pull breast tissue from the axillary region to permit the nipple to go into profile

336.   How does a carcinoma react under compression compared to a cyst?

4^{84}

341
A

    1.   spicules around the periphery disappear

    2.   more rigid

    3.   less distensible

    a.   1 and 2 only

    b.   1 and 3 only

    c.   2 and 3 only

    d.   1, 2, & 3

1⁸⁵ 337. Which of the following apply to coned down spot compression positioning?

1. vigorous compression is required
2. region of concern must be as close to the image receptor as possible
3. field size should be limited to the area of compression

a. 1 and 2 only
b. 1 and 3 only
c. 2 and 3 only
d. 1, 2, & 3

333
C

1⁸⁶ 338. Which of the following is appropriate when performing spot compression with magnification?

1. large focal spot
2. removal of the grid
3. increase to 30 kVp

a. 1 only
b. 2 only
c. 3 only
d. 1, 2, & 3

334
B

2⁸⁵ 339. What is the primary clinical indication for performing spot compression?

a. screening mammography
b. fatty breasts
c. it should be a routine procedure
d. to separate superimposed tissue

Mammography Techniques

```
┌─ Answer                                    Question # ─┐
│ ┌─ Question #                         Simulated Exam ─┐ │
│ │                                                    │ │
↓ ↓                                                    ↓ ↓
```

340.   With which of the following combinations should spot compression be used?   **2**^{86}

1.   non-grid
2.   magnification
3.   large focal spot

a.   1 and 2 only
b.   1 and 3 only
c.   2 and 3 only
d.   1, 2, & 3

^{344}
A

341.   What is the recommended focal spot size for magnification spot compression?   **3**^{85}

a.   0.1 - 0.2 mm
b.   0.4 - 0.6 mm
c.   0.8 - 1.0 mm
d.   1.2 - 1.5 mm

^{345}
A

^{346}
B

^{347}
D

136

3⁸⁶   342.   What is the primary characteristic of a carcinoma mass that requires vigorous compression to distinguish it from other masses?

    a.   a carcinoma will distort under compression
    b.   a carcinoma will move in relationship to other structures under compression
    c.   a carcinoma will not flatten under compression to the extent that glandular tissue will
    d.   a carcinoma will not distort the architecture of the breast under compression

D ³³⁷

4⁸⁵   343.   Which of the following apply to coned down spot compression positioning?

    1.   vigorous compression is required
    2.   precise positioning is required
    3.   field size should be limited to the area of compression

    a.   1 and 2 only
    b.   1 and 3 only
    c.   2 and 3 only
    d.   1, 2, & 3

B ³³⁸

D ³³⁹

137

344. Which of the following apply to the use of spot compression? 4^{86}

   1. more compression is required
   2. less rotation is required for the MLO
   3. pectoral muscle tension is desirable

   a. 1 only
   b. 2 only
   c. 3 only
   d. 1, 2, & 3

B ^{351}

345. What is the recommended focal spot size for magnification? 1^{87}

   a. 0.1 - 0.2 mm
   b. 0.4 - 0.6 mm
   c. 0.8 - 1.0 mm
   d. 1.2 - 1.5 mm

346. What is the maximum recommended magnification factor for mammography? 1^{88}

D ^{352}

   a. 1.5 X
   b. 2.0 X
   c. 3.0 X
   d. 4.0 X

347. What is the primary rationale for performing magnification mammography? 1^{89}

   a. evaluation of fatty tissue
   b. increase image contrast
   c. reduce patient dose
   d. increase detail of calcifications

2⁸⁷ 348. What happens to the areas of sharpness and unsharpness around an object when a smaller focal spot is used during magnification mammography?

    a. sharpness increases, unsharpness increases

    b. sharpness increases, unsharpness decreases

    c. sharpness decreases, unsharpness increases

    d. sharpness decreases, unsharpness decreases

2⁸⁸ 349. What is the purpose of an air-gap during magnification mammography?

    C³⁴²

    a. reduce patient motion

    b. reduce scatter radiation

    c. increase image density

    d. decrease exposure time

2⁸⁹ 350. Which of the following image characteristics may be expected on a magnification mammogram?

    1. increased resolution

    2. increased contrast

    3. increased density

    D³⁴³

    a. 1 and 2 only

    b. 1 and 3 only

    c. 2 and 3 only

    d. 1, 2, & 3

351. When is magnification mammography indicated? 3^{87}

1. during needle biopsies
2. as a problem solving measure
3. as a screening routine

a. 1 only
b. 2 only
c. 3 only
d. 1, 2, & 3

B ^{355} 352. Which of the following apply to magnification mammography? 3^{88}

1. patient dose is increased
2. image detail is increased
3. image contrast is increased

C ^{356}

a. 1 and 2 only
b. 1 and 3 only
c. 2 and 3 only
d. 1, 2, & 3

A ^{357}

3^{89} 353.   Which of the following determines which position should be used for a magnified mammogram?

        a.   two positions at right angles to one another are required

        b.   the position that best demonstrated the lesion with routine positions should be used

        c.   all magnification studies should be performed in the CC, MLO, and axillary positions   B ^{348}

        d.   either an exaggerated CC lateral or a MLO should be performed

4^{87} 354.   Which of the following factors affect magnification?

        1.   object to image receptor distance   B ^{349}

        2.   focal spot size

        3.   focal spot to object distance

        a.   1 and 2 only

        b.   1 and 3 only

        c.   2 and 3 only

        d.   1, 2, & 3

A ^{350}

355. What's the primary effect of magnification on resolution with the use of a large focal spot?

4 ^{88}

1. increased magnification increases resolution
C ^{361}
2. increased magnification decreases resolution
3. decreased magnification decreases resolution

a. 1 only
b. 2 only
c. 3 only
d. 1, 2, & 3

356. Which of the following is most often helpful in evaluating the margins of lesions?

4 ^{89}

C ^{362}
a. exaggerated CC lateral
b. coat hanger technique
c. magnification technique
d. increasing density

357. Which of the following is an appropriate technical factor adjustment for a post mastectomy axillary position?

1 ^{90}

1. increase kVp
2. increase distance
3. decrease mAs

A ^{363}
a. 1 only
b. 2 only
c. 3 only
d. 1, 2, & 3

1⁹¹   358.   Which of the following describes the difference between adjacent areas of darkness on a mammogram?

     a.   density
     b.   contrast
     c.   detail
     d.   distortion

1⁹²   359.   Which of the following can be expected as a result of using an extended developer processing time (EDPT) procedure?

353
B

     1.   increased contrast
     2.   increased kVp levels
     3.   decreased patient dose

     a.   1 and 2 only
     b.   1 and 3 only
     c.   2 and 3 only
     d.   1, 2, & 3

2⁹⁰   360.   Which of the following can be expected as a result of using a faster intensifying screen?

354
D

     1.   increased contrast
     2.   increased kVp levels
     3.   decreased patient dose

     a.   1 and 2 only
     b.   1 and 3 only
     c.   2 and 3 only
     d.   1, 2, & 3

361. What is the function of an automatic exposure control or phototiming device?

2^{91}

    a.   reduce exposure time
    b.   permits falling load mA
    c.   terminates exposure time
    d.   decreased required kVp levels

366
D

362. What occurs if the automatic exposure control or phototiming device density is increased?

2^{92}

    1.   higher kVp is used
    2.   higher mA is used
    3.   longer time is used

    a.   1 only
    b.   2 only
    c.   3 only
    d.   1, 2, & 3

367
C

363. What is the function of an automatic exposure control or phototimer backup timer?

3^{90}

    1.   avoid patient overexposure
    2.   assure sufficient image density
    3.   avoid generator damage

    a.   1 only
    b.   2 only
    c.   3 only
    d.   1, 2, & 3

368
B

3⁹¹ 364. Which of the following positions cannot be accomplished with an automatic exposure control or phototimer?

1. exaggerated CC lateral
2. cleavage (valley view or double breast compressions)
3. oblique lateral (Cleopatra)

a. 1 only
b. 2 only
c. 3 only
d. 1, 2, & 3

B ³⁵⁸

3⁹² 365. If the ion chamber of the automatic exposure control or phototimer is made more sensitive, which of the following will result?

1. shorter exposure time
2. decreased image density
3. decreased patient dose

a. 1 and 2 only
b. 1 and 3 only
c. 2 and 3 only
d. 1, 2, & 3

B ³⁵⁹

B ³⁶⁰

366. Which of the following generator configurations will produce the highest effective kVp for a given kVp setting on the control unit?

   a. three phase, 12 pulse
   b. three phase, 6 pulse
   c. single phase, 2 pulse
   d. high frequency

4^{90}

A ^{372} 367. What occurs if the kVp is increased when using an automatic exposure control or phototiming device?

   a. higher mA is used
   b. lower mA is used
   c. shorter time is used
   d. longer time is used

4^{91}

368. Which of the following enhances mammographic contrast?

^{373}
A

   1. decreased tissue thickness
   2. increased kVp
   3. a higher ratio grid

   a. 1 and 2 only
   b. 1 and 3 only
   c. 2 and 3 only
   d. 1, 2, & 3

4^{92}

1⁹³   369.   On which side of the mammogram should right and left markers be placed?

   a.   axillary
   b.   sternal
   c.   clavicular
   d.   inframammary crease

2⁹³   370.   Where should the skin marker be placed to evaluate skin calcifications on a tangential position?

   a.   adjacent to the area
   b.   opposite the area
   c.   2 mm lateral to the area
   d.   2 mm superior to the area

364
B

3⁹³   371.   Which of the following should be indicated by mammographic markers?

   1.   position performed
   2.   right or left breast
   3.   tissue thickness

   a.   1 and 2 only
   b.   1 and 3 only
   c.   2 and 3 only
   d.   1, 2, & 3

365
D

372. Which of the following designations is required to indicate a 60° MLO?

C ^{377}

1. 60°
2. ML
3. O

a. 1 and 2 only
b. 1 and 3 only
c. 2 and 3 only
d. 1, 2, & 3

4 ^{93}

A ^{378} 373. Which of the following grids can be used in mammography?

1. 4:1
2. 5:1
3. 8:1

C ^{379}

a. 1 and 2 only
b. 1 and 3 only
c. 2 and 3 only
d. 1, 2, & 3

1 ^{94}

B ^{380}

1⁹⁵ 374. Which of the following is necessary to produce a satisfactory film after removing a grid?

1. decrease compression
2. increase exposure time
3. decrease mAs

a. 1 only
b. 2 only
c. 3 only
d. 1, 2, & 3

A ³⁶⁹

2⁹⁴ 375. Which of the following categories of breast tissue should be mammographed with a grid?

1. fibroglandular
2. difficult to compress
3. thick

a. 1 and 2 only
b. 1 and 3 only
c. 2 and 3 only
d. 1, 2, & 3

A ³⁷⁰

2⁹⁵ 376. Approximately what percentage of radiation reaching the film is scatter?

a. 10
b. 25
c. 50
d. 80

A ³⁷¹

377. What is the primary function of a grid? 3^{94}

   a.   increase image density
   b.   decrease image density
   c.   increase image contrast
   d.   decrease image contrast

378. Which of the following will increase scatter 3^{95}
      radiation to the film?

A^{384} a.   removing the grid
                 b.   using a higher ratio grid
                 c.   decreasing kVp
                 d.   decreasing exposure time

379. What is the most desirable interspace material 4^{94}
      for mammographic grids?

                 a.   aluminum
                 b.   plastic fiber
B^{385} c.   carbon fiber
                 d.   lead

380. How does a grid accomplish its purpose? 4^{95}

                 a.   by filtering out high energy photons
                 b.   by filtering out scattered photons
                 c.   by screening intensifying screen
                      phosphor light
                 d.   by attenuating the primary x-ray beam
B^{386}

1⁹⁶   381.   What are the two routine needle localization positions?

a.   CC and MLO
b.   CC and true lateral
c.   CC and axillary
d.   MLO and axillary

1⁹⁷   382.   What term describes two positions that achieve right angle views of each other?

374
C

a.   adjacent
b.   comparison
c.   orthogonal
d.   diagonal

2⁹⁶   383.   Which of the following are types of preoperative localizing needle-wires?

1.   Frank
2.   Kopans
3.   Seldinger

375
D

a.   1 and 2 only
b.   1 and 3 only
c.   2 and 3 only
d.   1, 2, & 3

376
D

Mammography Techniques

384. For a needle localization of an inferior breast lesion, which of the following approaches is acceptable?

2^{97}

1. inferior
2. medial
3. lateral

B^{390}

a. 1 only
b. 2 only
c. 3 only
d. 1, 2, & 3

385. Approximately how much 1% methylene blue in sterile solution should be injected into the properly placed localization needle?

3^{96}

a. 0.1 ml
b. 1.0 ml
A^{391} c. 5.0 ml
d. 10.0 ml

386. Approximately how much air is appropriate for injection into the properly placed localization needle prior to the injection of methylene blue?

3^{97}

a. 0.1 ml
b. 1.0 ml
c. 5.0 ml
d. 10.0 ml

A^{392}

4⁹⁶   387.   What is the purpose of injecting air into the properly placed localization needle?

a.   localization marker for the pathologist

b.   localization marker for the radiologist   B³⁸¹

c.   it decreases the toxicity of the methylene blue

d.   it increases the radiopacity of the methylene blue

4⁹⁷   388.   Which of the following is another technique for pre-operative breast lesion localization?   C³⁸²

a.   stereotactic computerization

b.   double-walled needle

c.   endoscopic camera

d.   thermography

1⁹⁸   389.   When should specimen radiography be performed?

a.   within 24 hours of surgery

b.   as soon as the patient is in the recovery room   A³⁸³

c.   before the surgical procedure is terminated

d.   during follow-up mammography

153

390.   Which of the following are appropriate for specimen radiography?

2^{98}

1.   magnification
2.   increased kVp
3.   collimation to specimen size

B 397

a.   1 and 2 only
b.   1 and 3 only
c.   2 and 3 only
d.   1, 2, & 3

391.   What is the purpose of a thread attached to a needle that is placed into the lesion within a specimen during radiography?

3^{98}

a.   marker for the pathologist
b.   marker for the radiologist
c.   pathway for the methylene blue
d.   rotational marker for the mammographer

C 398

392.   Which of the following is desirable for specimen radiography?

4^{98}

D 399

1.   low kVp
2.   magnification
3.   increased kVp

a.   1 and 2 only
b.   1 and 3 only
c.   2 and 3 only
d.   1, 2, & 3

1⁹⁹ 393. Which position or technique best evaluates calcifications to determine if they are in the breast parenchyma or skin?

    a.   coat hanger
    b.   roll (turn view)
    c.   tangential
    d.   axillary

1¹⁰⁰ 394. Which of the following tissue regions of the breast are superimposed on the CC position?
    B ³⁸⁷

    a.   superior over inferior
    b.   medial over lateral
    c.   inferior over superior
    d.   lateral over inferior

2⁹⁹ 395. Which position is most useful in locating a lesion medially-laterally from the nipple?
    A ³⁸⁸

    a.   tangential
    b.   axillary
    c.   CC
    d.   45° oblique

2¹⁰⁰ 396. Why is it important to localize surgical scars on the breast prior to mammography?
    C ³⁸⁹

    a.   because compression may reopen them
    b.   they can mimic calcifications
    c.   they can mimic carcinoma
    d.   they may assist in plotting quadrants

397.   Of the following, which technique is the most helpful in localizing very small calcifications?

3^{99}

    a.   spot compression
    b.   magnification
    c.   high kVp
    d.   needle localization

398.   Which of the following may simulate a small calcification?

3^{100}

    1.   milk
    2.   deodorant
    3.   talcum powder

    a.   1 and 2 only
    b.   1 and 3 only
    c.   2 and 3 only
    d.   1, 2, & 3

399.   Which position is most useful in locating a lesion superiorly-inferiorly from the nipple?

4^{99}

    a.   tangential
    b.   axillary
    c.   CC
    d.   45° oblique

4^{100} 400. Which of the following tissue regions of the breast are superimposed on the 45° oblique position?

    a.   superior over inferior
    b.   medial over lateral
    c.   inferior over superior
    d.   lateral over inferior

393
C

394
A

395
C

396
C

B^{400}

ANSWERS AND EXPLANATIONS

1. (A) The breasts of women exposed to radiation are less sensitive to radiation after the age of 35. **(Feig)**

2. (C) The incidence of naturally occurring breast cancers has been shown to double between age 40-50. **(Feig)**

3. (B) Shoe store fluoroscopy operators are not one of the four main sources of epidemiological data on the breast. The four sources of data are Japanese atomic bomb survivors, benign breast disease patients, tuberculosis patients, and contralateral post radiotherapy cancer. **(Anderson)**

4. (B) Post menopause estrogen replacement therapy does not increase the risk of breast cancer. The known risk factors are family history of breast cancer, early menarche with late menopause, and first pregnancy after age 30. **(Scanlon)**

5. (B) Americans, Canadians, and northern Europeans are prone to a higher incidence of breast cancer than Japanese or Mexicans. **(Scanlon)**

6. (B) The carcinogenic effect of ionizing radiation is believed to have a latency period of approximately 7-10 years, which persists for the life of the patient. To date, there has been no conclusive evidence of a genetic link to radiosensitivity. **(Feig)**

7. (A) High caloric intake does not appear to increase risk to breast cancer. High fat, high protein, and excessive alcohol consumption appear to increase the risk. **(Scanlon)**

8. (D) Educational level does not effect the risk of developing breast cancer. Economic, person, and environmental factors have all been demonstrated to have an effect. **(Scanlon)**

9. (B) American Cancer Society guidelines for mammography recommend a baseline mammogram between the age of 35-40. **(American College of Radiology, Scanlon)**

10. (B) American Cancer Society guidelines for mammography recommend mammography every 1-2 years for women between the ages of 40 and 49, depending on findings and physician recommendations. **(American College of Radiology, Scanlon)**

11. (A) American Cancer Society guidelines for mammography recommend annual mammography for women over age 50. (American College of Radiology, Scanlon)

12. (B) American Cancer Society guidelines for mammography recommend breast self-examination for postmenopausal women monthly on the first day of the month to form a consistent date. **(American College of Radiology, Scanlon)**

13. (C) The upper outer quadrant is the area of highest incidence of breast cancer. **anatomy (Mitchell)**

14. (C) Lumps or thickening are the most common signs of breast cancer. **(American College of Radiology, Scanlon)**

15. (C) Normally the approximate skin thickness of the breast is 1.5 mm. **anatomy (Mitchell)**

16. (A) Lactation unrelated to pregnancy is termed galactorrhea and may be due to many causes, most of which are associated with high normal or elevated prolactin levels.
galactorrhea (Mitchell)

17. (D) Skin retraction is a consequence of such fibrotic changes involving the ligaments of Cooper, which are properly known as the breast suspensory ligaments. **skin retraction (Mitchell)**

18. (A) Skin retraction includes a spectrum of changes from a small local dimpling of the skin to shrinkage of the entire breast. **skin retraction (Mitchell)**

19. (B) Breast cancer is the most common form of cancer among all ages of women. **breast carcinoma - age distribution (Mitchell)**

20. (A) A galactocele is a cystic dilation of the mammary gland that often occurs at the areola. It is often the result of obstruction during lactation. **galactocele (Mitchell)**

21. (A) Intraductal adenocarcinoma has the highest incidence of occurrence. **adenocarcinoma (Mitchell)**

22. (D) Cysts of variable sizes are found in the breasts of more than 50% of women. **cysts (Mitchell)**

23. (A) Lymphedema, arm shoulder stiffness, and general numbness are all potential post breast surgery complications. **surgery, lymphedema (U.S. Department of Health and Human Services, Mitchell)**

24. (A) A tumor of 5 cm or larger in size and/or when 20% of the axillary lymph nodes test positive, adjuvant radiotherapy is indicated. **adjuvant radiotherapy (Mitchell)**

25. (D) The possible radiation risk to the patient from mammography is determined in part by the mean glandular dose, the patient's age at the time of the initial examination, and the patient's age at the time of the follow up examination. **(Feig)**

26. (C) The approximate average glandular dose for a screening mammogram is 0.1 rad or less. **(Feig)**

27. (D) The degree of breast compression, breast size and adiposity, and the x-ray beam HVL energy all affect breast dose per projection. **dose (NCRP)**

28. (C) The current incidence of breast cancer among American females is increasing. **incidence (U.S. Department of Health and Human Services)**

29. (D) Living in urban areas is not a factor that increases the risk of breast cancer for women. Obesity, pregnancy after age 30, and a family history of breast cancer have all been shown to contribute to the risk factor. **risk (U.S. Department of Health and Human Services)**

30. (A) Affluence and the fat content in the diet are factors that have been shown to increase the incidence of breast cancer in American women. Although nulliparity has an effect, once children have been born the number of children appears to have no effect. **risk (HHS)**

31. (C) A low white blood cell count does not increase the probability of surviving breast cancer. A high white blood cell count increases the survival rate. Breast cancer is more aggressive in younger women, older women are more prone to develop it, and a high fat content diet increases the probability of developing it. **risk (HHS)**

32. (D) Approximately 70% of patients diagnosed with breast cancer exhibit none of the known risk factors. **risk (Scanlon)**

33. (A) The American Cancer Society recommends beginning monthly breast self examination at age 20. **self examination (U.S. Department of Health and Human Services, Mitchell)**

34. (C) The importance of breast self examination is stressed partly due to the fact that mammography will miss approximately 10-15% of all cancers. **self examination (U.S. Department of Health and Human Services, Mitchell)**

35. (C) The 2nd, 3rd, and 4th fingers provide the best breast self examination technique. **self examination (U.S. Department of Health and Human Services, Mitchell)**

36. (B) Because breast self examination involves the acquisition of a motor skill, the most effective method has been shown to be allowing women to practice on a life-like model. **breast self examination (U.S. Department of Health and Human Services, Mitchell)**

37. (C) A breast self examination of the tail of Spence is best accomplished with the arm raised over the head. **self examination (U.S. Department of Health and Human Services, Mitchell)**

38. (D) The vertical strip, spiral, and quadrant-by-quadrant are all acceptable methods of breast self examination. **self examination (U.S. Department of Health and Human Services, Mitchell)**

39. (D) The valid arguments against breast self examination are that it enhances the risk of future invasive studies, compliance is best from the age group least likely to develop cancer, and self discovered lesions are 80-90% benign. **self examination (U.S. Department of Health and Human Services, Mitchell)**

40. (A) An advantage to teaching breast self examination with a screening program is that interval cancers may be detected. **self examination (U.S. Department of Health and Human Services, Mitchell)**

41. (B) 7-10 days after the onset of menstruation is the best time to perform a breast self examination. **self examination (U.S. Department of Health and Human Services, Mitchell)**

42. (D) The patient's elbows flexed, hands behind head, with elbows as posterior as possible is the proper position of the patient's arms during the visual inspection as part of a breast self examination or a clinical examination. **self examination (U.S. Department of Health and Human Services, Mitchell)**

43. (D) Breast self examination screening does not cause delays in physician visits. However it is inferior to a professional examination, it is inferior to mammography, and it does produce primarily benign lesions. **self examination (U.S. Department of Health and Human Services, Mitchell)**

44. (A) One disadvantage of breast self examination is its potential for inaccuracy. **self examination (U.S. Department of Health and Human Services, Mitchell)**

45. (D) Ultrasonographic examination of the breast is capable of distinguishing benign from malignant lesions, avoids the use of ionizing radiation, and is painless. **ultrasound (U.S. Department of Health and Human Services, Mitchell, Egan, American Society of Radiologic Technologists)**

46.   (D) A wide needle breast biopsy is not a painless procedure. It does use a cutting core needle, local anesthetic, and can be an outpatient procedure. **biopsy (U.S. Department of Health and Human Services, Mitchell, Egan, American Society of Radiologic Technologists)**

47.   (D) Galactography is useful in diagnosing intraductal masses, intraductal papillomas, and occult carcinomas. **ductography, galactography (U.S. Department of Health and Human Services, Mitchell, Egan, American Society of Radiologic Technologists)**

48.   (D) Breast ultrasonography is not valid for evaluation of the fatty breast. It is useful for evaluation of multiple cysts, tumor detection, and differentiation between cysts and solid masses. **ultrasound (Bassett BREAST CANCER, Mitchell, Egan)**

49.   (B) A hole plate is not used to establish a sterile field during a breast needle biopsy. It is used to compress the breast, to provide a grid reference for guidance of the needle, and to provide a visual reference for needle localization on the mammographic image. **biopsy (Bassett BREAST CANCER, Mitchell, U.S. Department of Health and Human Services)**

50.   (A) Pneumocystography is used for cyst treatment. It is not considered valid for cyst diagnosis or localization or tumor detection. **biopsy (Bassett BREAST CANCER, Mitchell)**

51.   (C) Water based contrast media is injected through the blunt tip of the needle during galactography. **ductography, galactography (Bassett BREAST CANCER, Mitchell, Egan)**

52.   (A) Bronchography is most similar to galactography. **ductography, galactography (Bassett BREAST CANCER)**

53.   (A) There are breast ultrasonographic units that permit reconstructions in planes other than sagittal and with patients in prone or supine positions, depending on the particular unit. **ultrasound (U.S. Department of Health and Human Services, Mitchell, Egan, Bassett BREAST CANCER)**

54. (D) Surgical breast biopsy confirms needle biopsy results, provides conclusive diagnosis, and produces about 75% benign diagnosis. **biopsy (U.S. Department of Health and Human Services, American Society of Radiologic Technologists, Mitchell, Egan)**

55. (C) The purpose of a breast biopsy is occult lesion detection. **biopsy (Bassett BREAST CANCER, Egan, U.S. Department of Health and Human Services)**

56. (D) Galactography is capable of evaluating duct ectasia, endocrine changes, and fibrocystic changes. **ductography, galactography (U.S. Department of Health and Human Services, Mitchell, Bassett BREAST CANCER)**

57. (D) The lower inner quadrant (LIQ) is least likely to develop carcinoma. **localization (U.S. Department of Health and Human Services, NCRP)**

58. (A) Hours on a clock face are normally used to describe the smaller sections used to localize lesions of the breast. **localization (Bontrager, American Society of Radiologic Technologists, Mitchell)**

59. (B) Both the UIQ (upper inner) and UOQ (upper outer) quadrants could include a breast lesion determined to be in the 10 o'clock position depending on whether it is the right or left breast. The left breast would be UIQ and the right breast would be UOQ. **localization (Bontrager, American Society of Radiologic Technologists, Mitchell)**

60. (C) Both the UIQ (upper inner) and UOQ (upper outer) quadrants could include a breast lesion determined to be in the 2 o'clock position depending on whether it is the right or left breast. The right breast would be UIQ and the left breast would be UOQ. **localization (Bontrager, American Society of Radiologic Technologists, Mitchell)**

61.   (B) The upper inner quadrant (UIQ) includes a right breast lesion determined to be in the 2 o'clock position. **localization (Bontrager, American Society of Radiologic Technologists, Mitchell)**

62.   (C) The lower inner quadrant (LIQ) would include a left breast lesion determined to be in the 8 o'clock position. **localization (Bontrager, American Society of Radiologic Technologists, Mitchell)**

63.   (B) The quantity of glandular tissue is a factor that determines the incidence of occurrence of cancer. **localization (Bontrager, American Society of Radiologic Technologists, Mitchell)**

64.   (D) A lesion that is localized at 5 o'clock on the right breast would be located in the lower inner quadrant (LIQ). **localization (Bontrager, American Society of Radiologic Technologists, Mitchell)**

65.   (C) The visual inspection of the patient prior to mammography does not require that all deodorant be removed. It is necessary that all jewelry has been removed from the neck and torso, that a strong light is used, and that the patient is examined both seated and recumbent examination. **clinical breast examination, physical breast examination (Andolina, Wentz, Egan, American Society of Radiologic Technologists, Mitchell)**

66.   (B) Areolar size is important to note as part of the visual breast examination. **clinical breast examination, physical breast examination (Egan, American Society of Radiologic Technologists, Mitchell)**

67.   (A) Lymph nodes smaller than 1 cm do not require further evaluation. Fixed or hard nodes and a 1.5 cm node would all require further evaluation. **clinical breast examination, physical breast examination (Egan, American Society of Radiologic Technologists, Mitchell)**

68.   (A) Both talcum powder and deodorant are unacceptable immediately prior to mammography because of the probability of metallic materials affecting image quality. High fat content food has no bearing on mammography. **clinical breast examination, physical breast examination (Andolina, Wentz, Egan, American Society of Radiologic Technologists, Mitchell)**

69.   (D) Some of the anatomical anomalies that should be noted during a physical breast examination include supernummary nipples, aplasia, and nipple inversion. **clinical breast examination, physical breast examination (Egan, American Society of Radiologic Technologists, Mitchell)**

70.   (C) A skin mole should be noted as it can simulate a well circumscribed intramammary lesion. **clinical breast examination, physical breast examination (Egan, American Society of Radiologic Technologists, Mitchell)**

71.   (C) A recent surgical breast scar may simulate radial spiculations. **clinical breast examination, physical breast examination (Egan, American Society of Radiologic Technologists, Mitchell)**

72.   (A) Two reasons why deodorants should be removed prior to mammographic examination are because the residues can appear radiopaque and they can mimic micro-calcifications. Deodorant fumes can not begin premature film developing. **clinical breast examination, physical breast examination (Andolina, Wentz, Bassett MAMMOGRAPHY, Mitchell, Long)**

73.   (C) Hands on hips with breasts thrust forward is the proper position of the arms during clinical breast examination palpation. **clinical breast examination, physical breast examination (Bassett MAMMOGRAPHY, Mitchell, Long)**

74.   (C) The purpose of the technologist's physical examination of the breast is to supplement the clinical history. It is not intended for making medical diagnosis or as part of the screening examination. **clinical breast examination, physical breast examination (Bassett MAMMOGRAPHY, Mitchell, Long)**

75. (C) The technologist should stand at the patient's right side when examining the right breast. **clinical breast examination, physical breast examination (Bassett MAMMOGRAPHY, Mitchell, Long)**

76. (D) The visual inspection criteria for breast examination includes notation of scars, moles, and lumps. **clinical breast examination, physical breast examination (Bassett MAMMOGRAPHY, Mitchell, Long)**

77. (A) The best position for palpation of the lymph nodes that drain the breast area is with the patient erect and bend forward at the waist. **clinical breast examination, physical breast examination (Bassett MAMMOGRAPHY, Mitchell, Long)**

78. (B) Variable finger pressure is valuable for detecting deep breast lesions during physical examination. **clinical breast examination, physical breast examination (Bassett MAMMOGRAPHY, Mitchell, Long)**

79. (D) Areas of retraction, inverted nipples, and deviated nipples all become more prominent when the breast is examined with the hands behind the head **clinical breast examination, physical breast examination (Bassett MAMMOGRAPHY, Mitchell, Long)**

80. (C) It is recommended that heavy pendulous breasts be manually lifted to obtain a view of the underside. **clinical breast examination, physical breast examination (Bassett MAMMOGRAPHY, Mitchell, Long)**

81. (D) Density of the parenchyma should influence the length of the interval between screening. Patient age and family history also have influence on interval time. **patient factors (Andolina, Wentz, Egan, American Society of Radiologic Technologists, Mitchell)**

82. (D) Hypothalamic pituitary dysfunction, cystic changes, and the use of oral contraceptives are all causes of nipple discharge. **history (Mitchell)**

83.   (B) The radiographer does not have a responsibility to educate the patient on breast self examination, although it is common for the radiographer to be involved in this educational process. Image quality, reduction of patient anxiety, and clinical history are all part of the radiographer's responsibilities during mammography. **breast self examination (American Society of Radiologic Technologists)**

84.   (C) Lobulations and smooth margins are both characteristic of fibroadenomas. Micro-calcifications are not. **fiberadenoma (American Society of Radiologic Technologists)**

85.   (D) Patients may convey consent to perform an examination in writing, orally, or through implication. **patient consent (Gurley, Torres)**

86.   (A) The chest wall is a common site for first re-occurrence of breast cancer. **re-occurrence (U.S. Department of Health and Human Services, American Society of Radiologic Technologists)**

87.   (B) Women whose mothers or sisters have had premenopausal beast cancer have 2-3 times the risk of developing the disease. **risks (American Society of Radiologic Technologists, U.S. Department of Health and Human Services)**

88.   (B) Parity is important because increased risk of breast cancer has been shown in childless females over age 30 **risk (American Society of Radiologic Technologists, U.S. Department of Health and Human Services)**

89.   (C) Early menarche with late menopause has been identified as risk for breast cancer. **risk (American Society of Radiologic Technologists, U.S. Department of Health and Human Services)**

90.   (D) The size, shape, and contour of the breasts are all important visual changes that should be noted during the clinical history for mammography. **(American Society of Radiologic Technologists)**

91.   (D) Appropriate actions for a patient who reports nipple discharge include milking the breast, pumping the breast, and obtaining a pathology sample. **risk, history (Mitchell)**

92. (A) The patient can withdraw consent verbally at any time. It is not necessary to have any other conditions fulfilled. **patient consent (Gurley, Torres)**

93. (B) The appropriate force for compression of the breast is 25-40 pounds. **(American College of Radiology)**

94. (C) The anode-heel effect produces greater radiation exposure toward the cathode and less toward the anode. **anode-heel (Carlton, Bushong, Curry)**

95. (A) Improperly applied compression is the most common factor that affects image quality in mammography. **breast compression (American College of Radiology)**

96. (D) Timer accuracy is not a quarterly quality control test for mammographic equipment. kVp accuracy, linearity, and reproduceability are recommended quarterly. **quality control (Gray, Long)**

97. (D) Mammographic grids should have a minimum of 80 lines per inch. **(Fajardo)**

98. (B) The size of the primary beam field can be reduced and image resolution can be increased with a steep anode angle x-ray tube. **anode, x-ray tube (Carlton, Bushong, Curry)**

99. (C) Mammography units utilize focal spots between 0.1 and 0.6 mm with the range for standard units being 0.3 - 0.6 mm. Focal spots between 0.1 and 0.2 are considered magnification focal spots for mammography. **focal spot (NCRP)**

100. (D) The amount of compression obtained during mammography is dependent on several factors including compressibility of the breast, patient tolerance, and the pathology that may be present. **compression, breast compression (Long, American College of Radiology)**

101.	(C) Both characteristic scatter and photoelectric interactions assist in producing optimal mammographic images. Compton scatter occurs at energy levels that are generally above those used for mammography and when produced it causes reduced image quality. **x-ray interactions (Carlton, Bushong Curry)**

102.	(B) Inherent filtration is that filtration that is part of the structure of the x-ray tube. **filtration, inherent (Carlton, Bushong, Curry)**

103.	(C) A bathroom scale can effectively accomplish quality control measurement of the compression device on a dedicated mammography unit. **compression (American College of Radiology)**

104.	(A) 0.03 mm of molybdenum (Mb) is the appropriate amount of filtration that must be added to the inherent filtration of a mammography tube. **(NCRP)**

105.	(D) An aperture diaphragm, cylinder cone, and collimator can all be used to restrict the beam on a dedicated mammography unit. **beam restriction, collimation (Curry, Bushong, Carlton)**

106.	(C) The recommended focal-film distance for mammography is 55-65 cm (22-26"). **(Fajardo)**

107.	(D) The terms plate, paddle, and device are all used to describe the breast compression units. **compression (Long, Eisenberg, American College of Radiology)**

108.	(A) The compression paddle must remain parallel to the receptor tray when compression is applied. **compression (Andolina)**

109.	(B) The primary disadvantage of using a grid with mammographic equipment is that is causes an increase in radiation dose. **(Fajardo)**

110.	(A) A finer wire mesh and lower kVp are used for film-screen quality control tests of mammographic cassettes as compared to the same tests for diagnostic radiographic cassettes. **(American College of Radiology, Long, Gray)**

111. (B) Because molybdenum emits lower characteristic energy photons within a relatively uniform range of energies, it is an ideal anode target material for mammography tubes. **molybdenum, anode, x-ray tube (Carlton, Bushong, Curry)**

112. (C) The compression plate should be 90° to the chest wall. **(American College of Radiology)**

113. (B) Characteristic photons from molybdenum are either 17.9 or 19.5 keV, within the range of 17-20 keV. **filtration (NCRP, Carlton)**

114. (D) Proper compression is best achieved with the use of a rigid right angle compression device that does not have rounded or sloping edges. **breast compression, breast imaging (Eisenberg, American College of Radiology)**

115. (A) Both the kVp and mA are limited by the heat unit rating of the mammographic x-ray tube. The focal-film distance is not affected. **heat units, x-ray tube ratings (Carlton, Bushong, Curry, Fajardo)**

116. (B) Both raising and lowering and angling rotation (medial-lateral) tube and film motions are commonly available with a dedicated mammography unit in order to adapt the unit to variations in patient body habitus. **(Long, American Society of Radiologic Technologists)**

117. (C) The cathode-anode axis of the mammographic x-ray tube is most commonly parallel to the transverse and sagittal planes when the patient is facing the unit with the coronal plane at a right angle and the transverse plane parallel to the surface of the film. **positioning (American Society of Radiologic Technologists, Long)**

118. (B) The K edge absorption of molybdenum is 20 keV. **filters (NCRP, Fajardo)**

119. (D) A 5:1 or 4:1 grid ratio is recommended for mammography. **grids (Long, Fajardo)**

120. (D) Compression decreases variation in radiographic density of the breast by increasing uniformity, it increases separation of breast tissue by decreasing tissue overlap, and it increases geometric sharpness by decreasing the object to image receptor distance. **breast compression, breast imaging (Eisenberg, American College of Radiology)**

121. (A) Molybdenum is the recommended mammography x-ray tube target material. **target, focal spot (NCRP, Carlton, Bushong, CU)**

122. (B) Mammography units utilize focal spots between 0.1 and 0.6 mm with the range for magnification examinations being 0.1 - 0.2 mm. Focal spots between 0.3 and 0.6 are considered standard focal spots for mammography. **focal spot (NCRP)**

123. (B) Fine adjustment is the primary purpose of the manual compression control as compared to the foot pedal control on a dedicated mammography unit. **compression paddle (Long)**

124. (B) Both a star test pattern and a pinhole camera are acceptable for measuring focal spot size. **quality control, quality assurance (Gray, Carlton, Fajardo, Bushong, Curry, Long)**

125. (D) Desirable characteristics of a compression device include a straight edge along the patient surface, foot pedal operation, and automatic release upon exposure completion. **compression paddle (Long)**

126. (B) The actual focal spot is the physical area that is impacted by the electrons from the x-ray tube filament. The effective focal spot is the focal spot that is projected out of the tube toward the object being radiographed. The focal track is the circular area around a rotating anode that is impacted by the electrons. **focal spot (Carlton, Bushong, Curry)**

127. (A) Compression decreases radiation dose by decreasing the thickness of the breast. Compression increases image contrast by decreasing scatter radiation. Compression increases image resolution by decreasing motion through immobilization. **breast compression, breast imaging (American College of Radiology, EI)**

128. (A) The fact that inherent filtration is too high and the fact that the tungsten target does not produce sufficient low energy photons are valid reasons for not using a standard diagnostic radiographic unit for mammography. Most diagnostic units are capable of achieving appropriate focal-film distances for mammography. **filtration, anode, target, x-ray tube, characteristic photons, tungsten, molybdenum (Carlton, Bushong, NCRP)**

129. (B) The average breast will fully compress to approximately 4 cm. **compression (Long)**

130. (B) Three ion chambers are the minimum to accommodate different breast sizes with dedicated mammographic equipment. **(Fajardo)**

131. (C) 20-35 kVp is the recommended range for mammography according to the ARRT specifications for the mammography examination. The NCRP publication #85 recommends 22-26 kVp. **radiographic sharpness (NCRP, Carlton, Bushong)**

132. (C) Beryllium is used to form the low energy absorbing window of a mammographic x-ray tube. **beryllium, anode, x-ray tube (Carlton, Bushong, Curry)**

133. (A) The emulsion and the intensifying screen must be placed toward the patient. The breast is likewise toward the emulsion and screen. However, the patient and screen are not placed away from the emulsion. **film, intensifying screens, single-emulsion film (Bushong, Curry, Carlton, Fajardo, Long)**

134. (A) 28 kVp with the appropriate mAs to produce a film density between 0.70 and 0.80 measured over the mesh area near the chest wall side of the film. Previously an OD of 2.75 and 3.25 was recommended. **screen-film contact (American College of Radiology, Gray)**

135. (D) Unique characteristics of single emulsion-single screen combinations include reduced speed, increased detail, and decreased expense. **film-screen combinations (Carlton, Bushong, Cullinan, Long)**

136. (D) Dirt, air, and cassette warping are all potential causes of poor film-screen contact. **film-screen contact (Carlton, Bushong, Cullinan)**

137. (C) Reduced patient dose is the primary benefit of using faster film-screen combinations. **film screen combinations, intensifying screens (Carlton, Bushong, Curry, Cullinan)**

138. (D) Image contrast is affected by film characteristics, processing conditions, and by tissue absorption. **contrast (Long, Carlton, Curry, Bushong, Cullinan)**

139. (C) Cassettes of 18 x 24 and 24 x 30 cm are recommended for mammography. **(Fajardo)**

140. (D) Mammography cassettes are constructed with thin sides to permit the film edge to demonstrate the chest wall. **cassettes (Carlton)**

141. (B) The emulsion side of a single emulsion film has a dull surface while the non-emulsion side exhibits the shinny surface of the bare film base. **film (Carlton)**

142. (C) Photographic materials should be stored between 60-70° F. **film storage, chemical storage (Carlton, Bushong, Curry, American College of Radiology)**

143. (B) The recommended humidity level for photographic material storage is 30-60%. **film storage (Carlton, Bushong, Curry, American College of Radiology)**

144. (A) The layer of the intensifying screen closest to the x-ray film emulsion is the protective coating. **intensifying screens (Carlton, Bushong)**

145. (A) Of the steps given, two are critical for sensitometric procedure accuracy. They are inserting the less exposed end of the sensitometric strip into the processor first and inserting all sensitometric strips on the same side of the processor feed tray. The sensitometric strip should be processed immediately after exposing, with no delay. **sensitometry, processing, quality control (Gray, Carlton, American College of Radiology, Bushong)**

146. (C) An optical density (OD) number of 1.25 is within the range recommended as the speed step (also known as the speed index or mid density) for sensitometric charting. Previously an OD of 1.20 was recommended. The actual determination of the speed step is OD 1.00 + base + fog, which is often within the range of 1.18 - 1.20 for a properly functioning film processor. **sensitometry, processing, quality control (Gray, Carlton, American College of Radiology, Bushong)**

147. (B) It is recommended that the mammography darkroom be cleaned daily. This should include mopping the floor at the beginning of the day and cleaning countertops with lint-free towels. **(American College of Radiology)**

148. (D) A retake or reject analysis can assist in reducing cost and patient exposures as well as evaluating the causes of repeated exposures. **repeat film studies (Carlton, Gray)**

149. (D) Both density and contrast would decrease as a result of insufficient replenishment occurring due to a quantity of large size films being run with the replenishment set for an average size film. **quality control, quality assurance (Gray, Carlton)**

150. (B) An artifact is an undesirable marking on a mammogram produced by handling, storage, or processing. **artifact (Cullinan, Bushong)**

151. (C) A sensitometer is used to produce an optical step wedge on a film for sensitometric measurement procedures. **sensitometry, processor quality control (Carlton, Gray, Bushong, American College of Radiology)**

152. (D) The type of filter, wattage of the light source, and the distance of the light from the film loading surface all affect the amount of safelight illumination in a darkroom. **safelight (Carlton, Bushong, Cullinan)**

153. (D) Pi lines occur at 3.14 x the circumference of the entrance roller of the processor. They occur when chemical deposits at the water level become significant while the processor is not operating. The deposits are then pressed into the soft film emulsion every time the roller turns on the film as it is processed. **artifact (Cullinan, Bushong)**

154. (C) A broken mercury thermometer could permanently contaminate a processor tank. Mercury does measure temperatures accurately and it does not coagulate easily. **film processing, processor, processor monitoring (Gray, Carlton, Bushong)**

155. (A) High darkroom humidity can cause water condensation on films which produces water droplet artifacts. Static artifacts are more easily produced when humidity is low. Half moon artifacts are caused by bending film during handling. **artifacts, film handling, processing temperature and humidity (Andolina, Wentz, Curry, Carlton, Bushong)**

156. (B) Most pressure artifacts are caused by the processor transport system. **film processors, processors, automatic processing (Carlton, Andolina, Wentz, Cullinan, Bushong, Gray)**

157. (D) Exposure factors, positioning, and wasted films should all be recorded during a retake/reject analysis. **(Carlton, Gray, Andolina, Wentz)**

158. (B) Accreditation phantoms are designed to consider the average compressed breast at 4.5 cm. or within a range of 4-5 cm. **phantom, quality assurance (Andolina, Wentz, American College of Radiology)**

159. (A) Developer underreplenishment causes both decreased image density and decreased image contrast. Fixer contamination is not a problem. **(Andolina, Wentz, Carlton, Bushong, Gray)**

160. (B) According to the American College of Radiology, at least 250 patients are required for a meaningful data base on which to base a mammographic film repeat or reject study. **repeat analysis (American College of Radiology)**

161. (C) Small areas of poor film-screen contact that remain after careful cleaning of the screen to remove dirt usually indicate that the foam backing behind the screen, which serves as a pressure plate, needs replacing. When the foam is replaced, the screen must also be replaced as separating the two usually damages the screen. **screen-film contact (American College of Radiology)**

162. (D) 2.0% difference between the primary x-ray beam field and the collimator light field is permissible during quality control testing of the field-to-light accuracy. **alignment, quality control, collimator (Carlton, American College of Radiology, Andolina, Wentz, Gray)**

163. (B) A non-dedicated film processing unit that is used for mammographic films may cause quality control problems due to volume fluxuations that cause the developer solution to become hyperactive or hypoactive and decreased image contrast. A non-dedicated film processing system will often exhibit decreased image noise, which is desirable, not a problem. **processing (Andolina, Wentz)**

164. (B) The frequency of intensifying screen cleaning is determined by the environment and usage but should be carried out at least weekly. **intensifying screens (American College of Radiology, Andolina, Wentz, Cullinan, Carlton, Gray)**

165. (A) Long cycle time processors that do not properly remove developer chemistry from the film can permit a dripping, curtain-like edge that is known as a curtain effect artifact. **artifact, film processing (Carlton, Curry, Bushong, Gray)**

166. (D) The darkroom fog level, viewboxes, and compression device should be checked regularly as part of a total mammographic quality control program. **(Andolina, Wentz, American College of Radiology)**

167.   (D) Increased contrast, reduced radiation dose, and increased tube life are all valid justifications for the use of extended mammographic film processing. **processing (Andolina, Wentz)**

168.   (B) Low darkroom humidity can cause static artifacts. High humidity can cause water condensation on films which produces water droplet artifacts. Half moon artifacts are caused by bending film during handling. **artifacts, film handling, processing temperature and humidity (Andolina, Wentz, Curry, Carlton, Bushong)**

169.   (D) Accreditation phantom images must be produced at 28 kVp. **phantom (American College of Radiology)**

170.   (C) Viewbox fluorescent tubes should be replaced approximately every 18-24 months. **(American College of Radiology)**

171.   (B) Accreditation phantom image scores permit comparative quality control to occur by matching new scores with older ones to evaluate the quality trends of the entire imaging system. **phantom, quality assurance (Andolina, Wentz, American College of Radiology)**

172.   (A) Developer measurements should be taken directly from the processor tank, not from the processor's digital or analog temperature display. **processing, processor monitoring (American College of Radiology, Andolina, Wentz, Carlton, Gray)**

173.   (A) Opaque foreign bodies prevent light from the intensifying screen from reaching the film thus creating an area of decreased density (a light area on the film). **artifact (Cullinan, Bushong)**

174.   (A) A densitometer is used to measure the optical density readings for sensitometric measurement procedures from an optical step wedge produced by a sensitometer on a film. **sensitometry, processor quality control (Carlton, Gray, Bushong, American College of Radiology)**

175. (D) Film fogging can be caused by exposure to light, improper safelight conditions, exposure to ionizing radiation, storage of film at high temperatures or humidity, and the use of film after the expiration date. **artifact, film handling (Cullinan, Carlton, Bushong)**

176. (B) Film is approximately twice as sensitive after exposure as before. **darkroom (Carlton, Cullinan)**

177. (A) The skin covering the breast is normally thickest at the base (about 2 mm compared to 0.5 mm at the nipple where it is normally thinnest). **(Andolina, Wentz, Mitchell)**

178. (B) Most of the glandular tissue is situated in the upper outer quadrants of the breast. **anatomy (Andolina, Wentz, Mitchell)**

179. (A) Cooper's ligaments are the thin fascial bands which support the breast. **anatomy (Mitchell, Andolina, Wentz)**

180. (C) 15-20 radially arranged lobes converge at the nipple. **anatomy (Mitchell, Andolina, Wentz)**

181. (B) Alveolar lobes empty onto the nipple through about 15-20 lactiferous ducts. **anatomy (Akesson, Mitchell, Andolina, Wentz)**

182. (C) The lactiferous sinus connects the alveolar lobes to the lactiferous ducts. **anatomy (Akesson, Mitchell, Andolina, Wentz)**

183. (D) Suspensory ligaments (Cooper's ligaments) are thin fascial bands that support the breast. **anatomy (Akesson, Mitchell, Andolina, Wentz)**

184. (A) The ampulla lies just below the areola. It is an area used for milk storage during lactation. **anatomy (Andolina, Wentz, Mitchell)**

185. (B) The junction between the inferior part of the breast and the anterior chest wall is termed the inframammary crease. **anatomy (Akesson, Mitchell, Andolina, Wentz)**

186. (A) The arterial supply for the breast is from the lateral thoracic artery, which is a branch of the axillary artery. **anatomy (Akesson, Mitchell, Andolina, Wentz)**

187. (B) The nipple is made primary of erectile tissue. **anatomy (Akesson, Mitchell, Andolina, Wentz)**

188. (A) Each breast is cone shaped with the base of the breast overlying the pectoralis major muscle. **anatomy (Akesson, Andolina, Wentz, Ballinger)**

189. (A) Breast lobules tend to decrease in size and number with increasing age, particularly after pregnancy. **anatomy (Akesson, Ballinger, Andolina, Wentz)**

190. (C) The breast parenchyma consists of glandular tissue (lobes and ducts). **anatomy (Akesson, Ballinger, Andolina, Wentz)**

191. (A) The breast stroma consists of adipose and connective tissue. **anatomy (Akesson, Ballinger, Andolina, Wentz)**

192. (D) The lateral thoracic branch of the axillary artery, the intercostal arteries, and the branches of the internal mammary artery all supply the breast. **arteries (Mitchell)**

193. (A) The pectoral subgroup is represented by #4. The lateral half of the breast drains mainly into the pectoral, apical, and subscapular subgroups of the axillary lymphatic nodes. **lymphatics, lymphatic drainage (Mitchell, Akesson)**

194. (C) The apical subgroup is represented by #1. The lateral half of the breast drains mainly into the pectoral, apical, and subscapular subgroups of the axillary lymphatic nodes. **lymphatics, lymphatic drainage (Mitchell, Akesson)**

195. (A) The small saccular gland or acinus is the milk producing unit of the breast. **anatomy (American Society of Radiologic Technologists, Ballinger, Andolina, Wentz)**

196. (D) The veins follow a similar pattern to the arteries. The axillary, intercostal, and internal mammary all supply venous drainage for the breast. **veins (Mitchell)**

197. (C) The axillary nodes vary in number from 12 to 30, or occasionally more. **anatomy (Eisenberg, Ballinger)**

198. (C) The nipple-areolar complex is supplied by the 4th lateral intercostal nerve and its branches. **nerves (Mitchell)**

199. (B) The retromammary space consists of adipose tissue which lies between the posterior aspect of the glandular tissue and the anterior aspect of the pectoral muscle. **anatomy (Ballinger, Andolina, Wentz)**

200. (A) The pectoralis minor lies posterior to the pectoralis major from the 3rd to 5th ribs. **anatomy, pectoral muscle (Ballinger, Akesson)**

201. (A) The postpubertal adolescent breast consists of primary dense connective tissue and casts a relatively homogeneous radiographic shadow with little tissue differentiation. **anatomy (Ballinger, Andolina, Wentz)**

202. (B) The retromammary space lies anterior to the pectoral major muscle and contains mostly adipose tissue. **anatomy (Ballinger, Andolina, Wentz)**

203. (C) A menopausal stage breast is represented by #3 in Figure 6. In the menopausal breast the glandular and stromal tissues undergo gradual atrophy. **anatomy (Andolina, Wentz, Ballinger, Bontrager, Mitchell)**

204. (D) A senescent stage breast is represented by #4 in Figure 6. In the senescent breast the menopausal changes continue to cause atrophy of the glandular and stromal tissues. **anatomy (Andolina, Wentz, Ballinger, Bontrager, Mitchell)**

205. (A) A pre-pregnancy stage breast is represented by #1 in Figure 6. The pre-pregnancy breast is composed primarily of dense connective tissue. **anatomy (Andolina, Wentz, Ballinger, Bontrager, Mitchell)**

206. (B) Colostrum is the milk-like fluid that is secreted by the breasts during pregnancy. Within a few days following birth it changes to milk. **anatomy, pregnancy (Akesson, Hole, Andolina, Wentz)**

207. (B) The lateral group of nodes is located lateral to the axillary artery near the lower border of the teres major muscle. **lymphatics, lymph nodes (Mitchell, Akesson, Andolina, Wentz)**

208. (D) Fibrous, glandular, and adipose tissue are the three major types of breast tissue. **anatomy, tissue (Bontrager, Andolina, Wentz, Mitchell)**

209. (B) Adipose tissue is less dense and connective tissue is more dense. Glandular tissue is more dense, not less. **anatomy, tissue (Bontrager, Andolina, Wentz)**

210. (D) Age, number of pregnancies, and hormone status as well as the inherent breast characteristics all affect the relative density of the breast tissue. **anatomy (Bontrager, Ballinger, Andolina, Wentz, Mitchell)**

211. (C) The embryologic origin of the female breasts is a well-differentiated apocrine sweat gland of the same type found in the axilla and elsewhere in the body. **anatomy (Andolina, Wentz)**

212. (A) Male breasts and the breasts of females over age 50 are composed primarily of fatty tissue. **anatomy (Andolina, Wentz, Bontrager, Mitchell)**

213. (A) Childless females over age 30 and females between age 15 and 30 would be expected to exhibit fibro-glandular breasts. **anatomy (Andolina, Wentz, Bontrager, Mitchell)**

214. (D) The distribution of fibrous connective tissue and ducts is accurately described as irregularly superimposed throughout the breast, the trabeculae arise from the broad base of the chest wall, and the connective tissue and ducts are located between the superficial and deep layers of superficial fascia. **anatomy (Andolina, Wentz, Egan, Mitchell)**

215. (A) Childbearing and advancing age causes glandular tissue to atrophy. **anatomy (Egan, Mitchell, Andolina, Wentz)**

216. (C) Females with 3 or more pregnancies would be expected to exhibit fibro-fatty breasts. **anatomy (Andolina, Wentz, Bontrager, Mitchell)**

217. (A) Involution is a retrograde change of the body or in a particular organ as in the changes in the female organs after pregnancy. **anatomy, physiology (Andolina, Wentz, Hole, Mitchell)**

218. (D) Many hormones, including insulin, growth hormone, corticosteroids, thyroxine, and human placental lactogen play important roles in breast development and lactation. **lactation (Mitchell, Andolina, Wentz)**

219. (C) Greater compression may be tolerated by decreasing breast sensitivity through decreasing caffeine intake 2 weeks prior to mammography and by performing mammography during the week after menses. Deodorant use should be avoided to prevent microcalcification artifacts. **physiology (Andolina, Wentz)**

220. (B) Normal changes as a result of the onset of menstruation include regression of the lobules and involution of the terminal ductal lobular unit. Replacement of parenchymal tissue by fat is a normal change following pregnancy and lactation. **physiology (Andolina, Wentz)**

221. (B) The atrophy of mammary structures that commences at menopause takes about 3-5 years to complete. **physiology (Andolina, Wentz)**

222. (B) Estrogen is responsible for ductal proliferation. **physiology (Andolina, Wentz)**

223. (C) Fatty tissue replaces supportive tissue in the involuting breast. **physiology (Andolina, Wentz)**

224. (C) Nursing the baby is desirable when mammography must be performed on the lactating breast because the removal of superimposed milk increases tissue visualization. **physiology (Andolina, Wentz)**

225. (D) The nipple region is the last to undergo menopausal involution. **physiology (Andolina, Wentz)**

226. (A) Normal results of involution include pendulous breasts and benign fatty lumps. Lobular proliferation occurs during pregnancy and lactation. **physiology (Andolina, Wentz)**

227. (B) The medial and posterior portions of the breast begin to atrophy first at menopause. **physiology (Andolina, Wentz)**

228. (A) Progesterone is responsible for lobular proliferation and growth. **physiology (Andolina, Wentz)**

229. (D) Adenosis, apocrine metaplasia (apocrine change), and sebaceous cysts are all benign diseases of the breast. **pathology (Andolina, Wentz, Mitchell)**

230. (C) Fibroadenomas are the most common benign breast neoplasms. It is estimated that 10-25% of women have one or more of these tumors. **pathology (Mitchell)**

231. (D) Nipple discharges that are persistent or nonlactational or unilateral are of clinical significance. **pathology (Andolina, Wentz, Mitchell)**

232. (A) The three primary presentations of mammographic pathology are masses, calcifications, and diffuse accentuation of the glandular tissues. **pathology (Andolina, Wentz)**

233. (C) Architectural distortion is the interruption of the natural flow of structures towards the nipple. **pathology (Andolina, Wentz)**

234. (A) Ductal adenocarcinoma is the most common type of breast carcinoma. This type rarely manifests any symptoms and by the time patients seek medical advice the tumor is usually in the infiltrative stage. **pathology (Mitchell, Andolina, Wentz)**

235. (D) A lipoma often presents as a radiolucent, encapsulated, and easily moveable mass. It is a fatty tumor with no epithelial component. **pathology (Andolina, Wentz, Mitchell)**

236.   (C) Approximately 40-50% of calcifications represent malignant breast disease. **pathology, malignancy (Andolina, Wentz, Mitchell)**

237.   (D) Carcinoma, obstruction of the lymphatics, and inflammatory disease are all potential causes of edema of the breast. **pathology (Andolina, Wentz, Mitchell)**

238.   (B) Mammographic characteristics of calcifications that are usually indications of malignant disease include varying densities and unilateral appearance. A calcification with a well defined border is more likely to be benign. **pathology, malignant (Andolina, Wentz, Mitchell)**

239.   (D) Arterial, popcorn type, and rim calcifications are usually benign. **pathology, benign (Andolina, Wentz, Mitchell)**

240.   (A) Secondary features of breast malignancy include skin thickening and/or retraction and axillary lymph node enlargement. When more than two discreet masses are detected they are usually benign. **pathology, malignancy (Mitchell)**

241.   (A) Micro-calcifications are often the only early sign of malignancy. **pathology, malignancy (Andolina, Wentz, Mitchell)**

242.   (A) An infiltrating carcinoma of the breast is often extremely hard on palpation and is larger on palpation than the mammographic image. A mass with an oval configuration and smooth margin is characteristic of a cyst. **pathology, malignancy (Mitchell)**

243.   (A) The primary signs that mammographic masses that are malignant are that they appear dense and have irregular margins. **pathology, malignancy (Mitchell)**

244.   (A) Calcifications that are new or have increased in number usually require biopsy. **pathology, malignancy (Mitchell)**

245.   (A) Thickened and dried secretions and necrosis are common causes of breast calcifications. **pathology, malignancy (Andolina, Wentz, Mitchell)**

246.   (C) The three primary presentations of mammographic pathology are masses, calcifications, and diffuse accentuation of the glandular tissues. **pathology, malignancy (Andolina, Wentz)**

247.   (D) Breast cysts are most common during menopausal years. **pneumocystography (Mitchell)**

248.   (D) The distribution, surrounding tissue or associated mass, and density of calcifications should be considered in determining whether they should be biopsied. In addition, shape, definition, unilateral or bilateral, increases in number, and size should be considered. **pathology (Andolina, Wentz)**

249.   (C) The CC position visualizes the central, subareolar, and medial portions of the breast. **positioning (American Society of Radiologic Technologists, Andolina, Wentz, Long)**

250.   (B) The CC position visualizes the central, subareolar, and medial breast tissue. The MLO does not visualize the medial region. **positioning (American Society of Radiologic Technologists, Andolina, Wentz, Long)**

251.   (A) When positioning for a CC position, the opposing arm should be brought forward and should hold onto the handle bar when one is available. **positioning (American Society of Radiologic Technologists, Andolina, Wentz, Long)**

252.   (C) When positioning for a CC position, the arm on the side of the body being imaged should be relaxed and externally rotated. **positioning (American Society of Radiologic Technologists, Andolina, Wentz, Long)**

253.   (C) The image receptor tray should be elevated to meet the edge of the elevated inframammary crease. This will cause the medial breast tissue to form a 90° angle to the chest wall. **positioning (American Society of Radiologic Technologists, Andolina, Wentz, Long)**

254.   (B) When properly compressed, the superior posterior portion of the breast is not imaged on the CC position. **positioning (American Society of Radiologic Technologists, Andolina, Wentz, Long)**

255.   (D) During the CC position the patient's head should be turned away from the side of interest. **positioning (American Society of Radiologic Technologists, Andolina, Wentz, Long)**

256.   (A) The axillary area is not visualized on the CC position. **positioning (American Society of Radiologic Technologists, Andolina, Wentz, Long)**

257.   (C) When the breast is positioned correctly for the CC position, but the nipple is not in profile an additional position should be obtained for the anterior breast only with the nipple in profile. **positioning (American Society of Radiologic Technologists, Andolina, Wentz, Long)**

258.   (B) The recommended procedure to remove wrinkling of the skin surface in the axillary area when positioning for a CC position is to place the arm of the affected side in a different position. **positioning (American Society of Radiologic Technologists, Andolina, Wentz, Long)**

259.   (D) Placing the opposite breast on the image receptor will insure the inclusion of all medial tissue during the CC position. **positioning (American Society of Radiologic Technologists)**

260.   (B) The CC and MLO positions are routine for screening mammography. **positioning (American Society of Radiologic Technologists, Andolina, Wentz, Long)**

261.   (A) A caudal-cephalic position is the recommended solution to performing the CC position on a kyphotic patient. **positioning (American Society of Radiologic Technologists, Andolina, Wentz, Long)**

262.   (A) Externally rotating the shoulder will usually remove the fat fold in the axillary area for a CC position. **positioning (American Society of Radiologic Technologists, Andolina, Wentz, Long)**

263. (C) The patient should stand 1/2 step back and lean in toward the image receptor tray for the CC position. **positioning (American Society of Radiologic Technologists, Andolina, Wentz, Long)**

264. (A) The pectoral muscle is visualized on the CC position occasionally. **positioning (Andolina, Wentz, Long)**

265. (A) The posterior medial area of the breast is not usually visualized on the MLO position. **positioning (Andolina, Wentz, Long)**

266. (D) The purpose of the MLO position is to, along with the CC position, provide the primary screening mammography position, to visualize as much of the axillary tail as possible, and, with the CC position, to permit visualization of lesions in two planes. **positioning (American Society of Radiologic Technologists, Andolina, Wentz)**

267. (A) The axis of the plane of compression is referred to when discussing obliques of the breast for the MLO position. **positioning (Long, Andolina, Wentz)**

268. (A) The MLO demonstrates more tissue than any other position. **positioning (Andolina, Wentz, Long)**

269. (B) The x-ray tube should be positioned parallel to the pectoral muscle when positioning for a MLO position. **positioning (American Society of Radiologic Technologists, Andolina, Wentz, Long)**

270. (A) The upper outer quadrant is best visualized with a MLO position. **positioning (American College of Radiology, Andolina, Wentz, Long)**

271. (D) 60° is the approximate recommended tube angle for a MLO position of an asthenic patient. **positioning (Andolina, Wentz, Long)**

272. (B) The MLO position demonstrates the pectoral muscle to the nipple as well as the inframammary crease. **positioning (American Society of Radiologic Technologists, Andolina, Wentz, Long)**

273. (A) To demonstrate as much of the pectoralis muscle as possible the patient should rotate the shoulder anteriorly immediately prior to final compression for the MLO position. **positioning (American Society of Radiologic Technologists, Andolina, Wentz, Long)**

274. (B) Pectoralis excavatum is a condition characterized by a depressed sternum. It presents severe problems in obtaining a satisfactory MLO position of the breast. **positioning (Long, Andolina, Wentz)**

275. (B) The breast tissue and pectoralis muscle should be moved anterior and lateral when positioning the breast for a MLO position. **positioning (American Society of Radiologic Technologists, Andolina, Wentz, Long)**

276. (D) A line drawn from the shoulder to mid-sternum will determine the correct tube angle for a MLO position. **positioning (Andolina, Wentz, Long)**

277. (B) A small quantity of tissue below the inframammary crease should be demonstrated on a MLO position to insure that the breast has been demonstrated to the chest wall. **positioning (Long, Andolina, Wentz)**

278. (A) The MLO position is preferred over the true lateral because of its effectiveness in visualizing both the posterior breast and the upper outer quadrant. **positioning (Andolina, Wentz, Long)**

279. (C) The arm of the affected side be placed forward to grasp the handlebar for a MLO position. **positioning (American Society of Radiologic Technologists)**

280. (B) Depending on the patient's body habitus, tube angles of 40-70° are used for the MLO position. **positioning (Long, Andolina, Wentz)**

281. (C) The cleavage position would best demonstrate an extreme medial lesion of the breast. **positioning (American Society of Radiologic Technologists, Long, Andolina, Wentz, Egan)**

282. (A) The primary reasons for performing a ML or LM 90° position of the breast are to provide identification of the exact location of a lesion in the sagittal plane and to demonstrate UIQ or LIQ tissue. The cleavage position is used to demonstrate a maximum quantity of medial tissue. **positioning (American Society of Radiologic Technologists, Andolina, Wentz, Long)**

283. (C) The LM or ML position best demonstrates the effect of gravity or air-fluid/fat levels in the breast. **positioning (American Society of Radiologic Technologists, Andolina, Wentz, Long)**

284. (C) The LM or ML 90° positions can be substituted for the MLO position for patients with pectoralis excavatum. **positioning (American Society of Radiologic Technologists, Andolina, Wentz, Long)**

285. (B) The coat hanger technique best demonstrates the remote tissue in the peripheral area of the breast, especially adjacent to the ribs. **positioning (American Society of Radiologic Technologists, Andolina, Wentz, Long)**

286. (C) A lesion is located in the medial portion of the breast if it appears higher on a 90° lateral as compared to the MLO position. **positioning (Egan, Andolina, Wentz, Long)**

287. (C) A 30° oblique position should be performed if a lesion is visualized on the MLO position but not on an exaggerated CC lateral. **positioning (Egan, Andolina, Wentz, Long)**

288. (B) The exaggerated CC lateral position is used to demonstrate tissue in the outer aspect of the breast that is not visualized on the routine CC position. **positioning (Long, Egan, Andolina, Wentz)**

289. (B) The LMO position is recommended for post-operative open heart surgery patients or patients with a prominent pacemaker. **positioning (American Society of Radiologic Technologists, Andolina, Wentz, Long, Egan)**

290. (D) A 70° angle would produce the best image of a right breast 1:00 lesion with a reverse LMO position. A 20° reverse LMO should be used for lesions of the right breast at 2:30 or 8:30 or left breast at 9:30 or 3:30. A 70° reverse LMO should be used for lesions of the right breast at 1:00 or 7:00 or left breast at 11:00 or 5:00. **positioning (American Society of Radiologic Technologists)**

291. (C) The roll or turn view is often useful to demonstrate tissue that has been superimposed on another position. **positioning (American Society of Radiologic Technologists, Andolina, Wentz, Long)**

292. (C) The ML 90° or LM 90°positions are most helpful in demonstrating tissue in the 12:00 or 6:00 position. **positioning (American Society of Radiologic Technologists)**

293. (A) The exaggerated CC lateral position best demonstrates tissue that extends just beyond the edge of the image receptor plate following the curve of the rib cage on the CC position. **positioning (American Society of Radiologic Technologists, Andolina, Wentz, Long)**

294. (C) The oblique lateral (Cleopatra) position best demonstrates deep axillary tissue. **positioning (Long, Andolina, Wentz)**

295. (B) Lesions seen in the upper inner or lower outer quadrant require a lateromedial (reverse) oblique angulation of some degree depending on the location of the lesion.

296. (C) The ML 90° or LM 90° positions should be performed to determine if a lesion is milk or calcium because they permit the milk to form a fluid level or teacup sign. **positioning (American Society of Radiologic Technologists, Egan, Andolina, Wentz)**

297. (C) The tangential position will project a questionable area in the breast as close as possible to the subcutaneous fat. **positioning (American Society of Radiologic Technologists, Egan, Long)**

298. (B) The roll or turn view is used to triangulate lesions. **positioning (American Society of Radiologic Technologists, Egan, Long)**

299. (D) The 30° oblique, exaggerated CC lateral, and oblique lateral (Cleopatra) positions are all designed to assist in enhancing UOQ lesions, where more carcinomas occur than any other region of the breast. **positioning (American Society of Radiologic Technologists, Andolina, Wentz, Long)**

300. (A) A 20° angle would produce the best image of a right breast 2:30 lesion with a reverse LMO position. A 20° reverse LMO should be used for lesions of the right breast at 2:30 or 8:30 or left breast at 9:30 or 3:30. A 70° reverse LMO should be used for lesions of the right breast at 1:00 or 7:00 or left breast at 11:00 or 5:00. **positioning (American Society of Radiologic Technologists)**

301. (D) The ML 90° or LM 90° position best demonstrates in a tangential position lesions in the superior or inferior breast regions best. **positioning (American Society of Radiologic Technologists, Andolina, Wentz, Long)**

302. (C) The cleavage position (also known as the valley view or double breast compressions position) best demonstrates tissue that extends over the sternum. **positioning (Andolina, Wentz, Long)**

303. (B) The breast tissue should be pulled superior and lateral (up and out) when positioning for a mediolateral lateral position. **positioning (Andolina, Wentz, American Society of Radiologic Technologists)**

304. (A) The primary objective of performing a 30° oblique position is to image the axillary tail and deep UOQ of the breast. **positioning (Andolina, Wentz, Long)**

305. (D) A lesion outside compressible breast tissue, a lesion very high on the chest wall, and a lesion very close to a silicone implant are all indications for the coat hanger technique. **positioning (Andolina, Wentz, Long)**

306. (A) When the patient does not straighten up, the C-arm should not be angled for the oblique lateral (Cleopatra) position. However, it is suggested that when possible, the C-arm should be angled to permit the patient to assume a more comfortable and erect position. **positioning (Andolina, Wentz, Long)**

307. (A) The CC position best demonstrates in a tangential view lesions in the medial or lateral breast regions best. **positioning (American Society of Radiologic Technologists, Andolina, Wentz, Long)**

308. (A) A 20° angle would produce the best image of a left breast 9:30 lesion with a reverse LMO position. A 20° reverse LMO should be used for lesions of the right breast at 2:30 or 8:30 or left breast at 9:30 or 3:30. A 70° reverse LMO should be used for lesions of the right breast at 1:00 or 7:00 or left breast at 11:00 or 5:00. **positioning (American Society of Radiologic Technologists)**

309. (A) Breast tissue should be displaced anteriorly when imaging the augmented breast with Eklund positioning. **positioning (Eklund, American College of Radiology, Andolina, Wentz, Long)**

310. (A) The axillary position is recommended for screening of post mastectomy patients. **positioning (American Society of Radiologic Technologists, Andolina, Wentz, Long)**

311. (B) The use of a spot compression paddle is a potential solution to the problem created by extremely small breasts that will not remain under compression. **positioning (Long, Andolina, Wentz)**

312. (C) The 90° lateral is recommended when the Eklund positions cannot be used to visualize the augmented breast. **positioning (Eklund, American College of Radiology, Andolina, Wentz, American Society of Radiologic Technologists, Long)**

313. (A) The axillary position best demonstrates recurring lesions along the chest wall of post mastectomy patients. **positioning (Long, Andolina, Wentz)**

314. (A) Both the routine CC and MLO and the modified Eklund CC and MLO are recommended for a complete study of the augmented breast. **positioning (Eklund, Long, American Society of Radiologic Technologists, Andolina, Wentz)**

315. (C) A CC and MLO position of the unaffected breast as well as an axillary position of the affected breast are required for a complete mammographic study of the unilateral post mastectomy breast. **positioning (Long, Andolina, Wentz)**

316. (D) The contraindications for performing Eklund positions of the augmented breast include when tissue is firmly encapsulated and cannot be displaced posteriorly, when little tissue is surrounding the implant, and for post mastectomy implants surrounded by skin only. **positioning (Eklund, American College of Radiology, Andolina, Wentz, Long)**

317. (A) The CC and MLO positions demonstrate the posterior tissue of the augmented breast. **positioning (Eklund, American Society of Radiologic Technologists, Andolina, Wentz, Long)**

318. (B) The lateromedial (reverse) oblique position is used to obtain tangential studies of lesions and as a third position of an encapsulated implant when the Eklund technique is not possible. The LM or ML 90° positions can be substituted for normal screening positions for patients with pectoralis excavatum. **positioning (American Society of Radiologic Technologists, Andolina, Wentz, Long)**

319. (D) Rationale for utilizing Eklund positions for mammography of the augmented breast include the fact that 2-5 cm of additional compression can be achieved, image detailed is enhanced by improved compression, and significantly more tissue is visualized. **positioning (Eklund, American Society of Radiologic Technologists, Andolina, Wentz, Long)**

320. (A) The axillary position can be performed on post mastectomy patients without compression while maintaining satisfactory quality of the mammogram. **positioning (Long, Andolina, Wentz)**

321. (C) Gripping the hand rail tightly will tighten the pectoral muscle, thus adding difficulty to positioning and compression. Although raising the shoulder may tighten the pectoral muscle, it is not as likely to cause positioning and compression problems. **positioning (Andolina, Wentz, Long)**

322. (C) Lesions at 6:00 or 12:00 within the breast will best be visualized with a true lateral position. Lesions at 3:00 on the left breast or 6:00 on the right breast will best be visualized with an exaggerated CC position. **positioning (Andolina, Wentz, Long)**

323. (A) The axillary position should be performed to demonstrate recurrences of carcinoma on the affected side of post mastectomy patients. **positioning (American Society of Radiologic Technologists, Andolina, Wentz, Long)**

324. (B) The prosthesis be displaced posteriorly and superiorly when positioning the augmented breast with Eklund positions. **positioning (Eklund, American College of Radiology, Andolina, Wentz, Long)**

325. (B) Breast tissue moves toward the nipple when compression is applied. **compression (American Society of Radiologic Technologists, Andolina, Wentz, Long)**

326. (B) The primary goal of compression is to uniformly reduce the thickness of the breast. **compression (American Society of Radiologic Technologists, Andolina, Wentz, Long)**

327. (B) The two true statements regarding the use of motorized foot control compression are that it leaves both hands free to position the breast and it should be used only during the first stage of compression. **compression (American Society of Radiologic Technologists, Andolina, Wentz, Long)**

328. (D) Good breast compression reduces object to film distance, separates internal structures for better visualization, and reduces scatter radiation to the image. **compression (American Society of Radiologic Technologists, Andolina, Wentz, American College of Radiology, Long, Carlton, BU)**

329. (C) The guideline for adequate compression is when breast tissue is firm and taut (tight) to the touch. **compression (American Society of Radiologic Technologists, Andolina, Wentz, Long)**

330. (A) A more homogenous film density is produced as a result of vigorous compression because the posterior and anterior tissue is spread to an even thickness. **compression (Long, Andolina, Wentz)**

331. (C) Vigorous compression permits more accurate evaluation of masses because cysts and normal glandular tissue are more easily compressed than carcinomas. **compression (Andolina, Wentz, Long)**

332. (B) Vigorous compression increases both image contrast and detail as compared to poor compression of the same breast. Image density is increased due to the decrease in tissue thickness. **compression (Andolina, Wentz, Long, Carlton, Bushong)**

333. (C) An adenosis describes the development of new lobular units or their enlargement. **adenosis (Andolina, Wentz, Eisenberg)**

334. (B) Spot and flat compression devices are acceptable for use with film-screen mammography. Curved compression was used for xeroradiography and is unacceptable for film-screen mammography. **compression (Andolina, Wentz)**

335. (A) It is important to avoid repositioning and sacrificing the demonstration of tissue in another direction. An additional position should be obtained of the anterior breast tissue with the nipple in profile. **compression (Andolina, Wentz, Long)**

336. (C) A carcinoma is more rigid and less distensible under compression than a cyst. **compression (Long, Andolina, Wentz)**

337. (D) When performing coned down spot compression positioning it is important to apply vigorous compression, move the region of concern as close to the image receptor as possible, and to limit the field size to the area of compression. **compression (Long, Andolina, Wentz)**

338. (B) Removal of the grid is appropriate when performing spot compression with magnification. In addition, the small focal spot should be used and the field should be coned down to the area of interest only. **compression (Long, Andolina, Wentz)**

339. (D) Spot compression is performed primarily to separate superimposed tissue. **compression (Long, Andolina, Wentz)**

340. (A) Spot compression should be used non-grid when used with magnification. In addition, a small focal spot should be used. **compression (Long, Andolina, Wentz)**

341. (A) A 0.1 - 0.2 mm focal spot size is recommended for magnification spot compression. **compression (Long, Andolina, Wentz)**

342. (C) The fact that a carcinoma will not flatten under compression to the extent that glandular tissue will is the primary characteristic that requires vigorous compression to distinguish it from other masses. **compression (Long, Andolina, Wentz)**

343. (D) When performing coned down spot compression positioning it is important to apply vigorous compression, limit the field size to the area of compression, and utilize precise positioning. **compression (Long, Andolina, Wentz)**

344. (A) More compression is required during spot compression than would be used for full breast compression. **compression (Long, Andolina, Wentz)**

345. (A) A 0.1 - 0.2 mm focal spot size is recommended for magnification. **magnification (Long, Andolina, Wentz, Carlton, Bushong, Curry)**

346. (B) 2.0 X is the maximum recommended magnification factor for mammography. **magnification (Long, Wentz)**

347. (D) The primary rationale for performing magnification mammography is to increase the detail of calcifications. **magnification (Long, AND)**

348. (B) Sharpness increases while unsharpness decreases around an object when a smaller focal spot is used during magnification mammography. **magnification (Long, Andolina, Wentz, Carlton, Bushong, Curry)**

349. (B) An air-gap during magnification mammography will decrease scatter radiation, thus improving image contrast. **air-gap, magnification (Long, Andolina, Wentz, Carlton, Bushong, Curry)**

350. (A) Magnification mammograms should exhibit increased resolution, increased contrast, and decreased image density. **magnification (Long, Andolina, Wentz, Carlton)**

351. (B) Magnification mammography is indicated as a problem solving measure only. **magnification (Long, Andolina, Wentz)**

352. (D) Patient dose as well as image detail and contrast are all increased during magnification mammography. **magnification (Long, Andolina, Wentz, Carlton, Bushong, Curry)**

353. (B) The position that best demonstrated the lesion with routine positions should be used for a magnified mammogram. **magnification (Long, AND)**

354. (D) Many factors affect magnification including object to image receptor distance, focal spot size, and focal spot to object distance. In addition, focal spot to image receptor distance has a direct effect. **size distortion, magnification (Carlton, Bushong, Curry)**

355. (B) Increased magnification decreases resolution if no other factors are changed. However, in magnification mammography a small focal spot permits magnification to increase the size of a small lesion without significantly changing (or even while increasing) the resolution or detail. **size distortion, magnification (Carlton, Bushong, Curry)**

356. (C) Magnification mammography is most often helpful in evaluating the margins of lesions because the increased size and detail makes visualization easier. **magnification (Long, Andolina, Wentz)**

357. (A) Increased kVp is required for a post mastectomy axillary position. **technique, exposure factors (American Society of Radiologic Technologists, Long, Andolina, Wentz)**

358. (B) Contrast is the difference between the areas of darkness on a mammogram. **contrast (Carlton, Long, Andolina, Wentz, Bushong)**

359. (B) Increased contrast and decreased patient dose can be expected as a result of using an extended developer processing time (EDPT) procedure. **extended developer processing time (EDPT) (Long, American College of Radiology, Andolina, Wentz)**

360. (B) Increased contrast and decreased patient dose can be expected as a result of using a faster intensifying screen. **intensifying screens (Carlton, Bushong, Curry, Long, Andolina, Wentz)**

361. (C) An automatic exposure control or phototiming device terminates the exposure time. **phototiming, automatic exposure control (Carlton, Cullinan, Bushong, Long, Andolina, Wentz, Curry)**

362. (C) If the automatic exposure control or phototiming device density is increased, the x-ray generator will use a longer exposure time. **phototiming, automatic exposure control (Carlton, Cullinan, Bushong, Long, Andolina, Wentz, Curry)**

363. (A) The functions of an automatic exposure control or phototimer backup timer are to avoid patient overexposure and protect the x-ray tube from overloading. **phototiming, automatic exposure control (Carlton, Cullinan, Bushong, Curry)**

364. (B) The cleavage (valley view or double breast compressions) position cannot be accomplished with an automatic exposure control or phototimer because there is no tissue placed over the ion chamber. **phototiming, automatic exposure control (Carlton, Cullinan, Bushong, Long, Andolina, Wentz, Curry)**

365. (D) If the ion chamber of the automatic exposure control or phototimer is made more sensitive, shorter exposure time, decreased image density, and decreased patient dose will all result. **phototiming, automatic exposure control (Carlton, Cullinan, Bushong, Long, Andolina, Wentz, Curry)**

366. (D) A high frequency generator configuration will produce the highest effective kVp for a given kVp setting on the control unit. In descending order from the highest effective kVp the other configurations are three phase, 12 pulse; three phase, 6 pulse; and single phase, 2 pulse. **generators, ripple (Carlton, Bushong, Andolina, Wentz, Curry)**

367. (C) If the kVp is increased when using an automatic exposure control or phototiming device a shorter time is used. **phototiming, automatic exposure control (Carlton, Cullinan, Bushong, Long, Andolina, Wentz, Curry)**

368. (B) Mammographic contrast is enhanced by decreased tissue thickness, decreased kVp, and a higher ratio grid. **contrast (Carlton, Long, Bushong)**

369. (A) Right and left markers should be placed on the axillary side of the mammogram. **markers (Long, American Society of Radiologic Technologists)**

370. (A) A skin marker should be placed adjacent to the skin calcifications for their evaluation on a tangential position. **markers (Long, American Society of Radiologic Technologists)**

371. (A) Both the position performed and right or left breast must be indicated by mammographic markers. **markers (Long, American Society of Radiologic Technologists)**

372. (A) The designations 60° and ML are required to indicate a 60° MLO. **markers (Long, Andolina, Wentz)**

373. (A) 4:1 and 5:1 ratio grids are used in mammography. An 8:1 grid is for diagnostic radiography. **grids (Andolina, Wentz, Long, Carlton, Bushong, Cullinan, Curry)**

374. (C) mAs must be reduced to produce a satisfactory film after removing a grid. **grids (Andolina, Wentz, Long, Carlton, Bushong, Cullinan, Curry)**

375. (D) Fibroglandular, difficult to compress breasts, and thick breast tissue should all be mammographed with a grid. **grids (Andolina, Wentz, Long, Carlton, Bushong, Cullinan, Curry)**

376. (D) Approximately 80-85% of the radiation reaching the film is estimated to be scatter. **grids (Andolina, Wentz, Long, Carlton, Bushong, Cullinan, Curry)**

377. (C) The primary function of a grid is to increase image contrast. **grids (Andolina, Wentz, Long, Carlton, Bushong, Cullinan, Curry)**

378. (A) Removing the grid will increase scatter radiation to the film. **grids (Andolina, Wentz, Long, Carlton, Bushong, Cullinan, Curry)**

379. (C) Carbon fiber is the best mammographic grid interspace material because it absorbs less of the primary beam than plastic or aluminum. **grids (Andolina, Wentz, Long, Carlton, Bushong, Cullinan, Curry)**

380. (B) A grid functions by filtering out scattered, lower energy photons. **grids (Andolina, Wentz, Long, Carlton, Bushong, Cullinan, Curry)**

381. (B) The two routine needle localization positions are the CC and true lateral. **localization (Long, Andolina, Wentz, Ballinger)**

382. (C) Orthogonal views are two positions that achieve right angle views of each other. **localization (Long, Andolina, Wentz, Ballinger)**

383. (A) The common types of preoperative localizing needle-wires include the Frank and Kopans needles. The Seldinger needle is used for arterial vascular punctures. Other types of preoperative localizing needle-wires include the Homer, Hawkins, Urrutia, and Sadowsky needles. **localization (Long, Andolina, Wentz, Ballinger)**

384. (A) For a needle localization of an inferior breast lesion, only an inferior approach is acceptable. **localization (Long, Andolina, Wentz, Ballinger)**

385. (B) Approximately 1 ml (cc) of 1% methylene blue in sterile solution should be injected into the properly placed localization needle. **localization (Long, Andolina, Wentz, Ballinger)**

386. (B) Approximately 1 ml (cc) of air is appropriate for injection into the properly placed localization needle prior to the injection of methylene blue. **localization (Long, Andolina, Wentz, Ballinger)**

387. (B) Air is injected into the properly placed localization needle as a marker for the radiologist when viewing the post needle placement mammograms. **localization (Long, Andolina, Wentz, Ballinger)**

388. (A) Stereotactic computerization is another technique for pre-operative breast lesion localization. **localization (Andolina, Wentz, Ballinger)**

389. (C) Specimen radiography should be performed while the patient is still undergoing surgery. **specimen radiography (Andolina, Wentz, Ballinger, Long)**

390. (B) Specimen radiography should be performed with magnification and with collimation to the specimen size. Increased kVp should not be used. **specimen radiography (Andolina, Wentz, Ballinger, Long)**

391. (A) A thread is attached to a needle that is placed into the lesion within a specimen during radiography as a marker for the pathologist. **specimen radiography (Andolina, Wentz, Ballinger, Long)**

392. (A) Low kVp and magnification are desirable for specimen radiography. **specimen radiography (Andolina, Wentz, Ballinger, Long)**

393. (C) The tangential position best evaluates calcifications to determine if they are in the breast parenchyma or skin. **localization (Andolina, Wentz, Ballinger)**

394. (A) The superior tissue region is superimposed over the inferior region of the breast by the CC position. **localization (Andolina, Wentz, Ballinger)**

395. (C) The CC position is most useful in locating a lesion medially-laterally from the nipple. **localization (Andolina, Wentz, Ballinger)**

396. (C) It is important to localize surgical scars on the breast prior to mammography because they can mimic carcinoma. **localization (Andolina, Wentz, Ballinger)**

397. (B) Magnification techniques are most helpful in localizing very small calcifications. **localization (Andolina, Wentz, Ballinger)**

398. (C) Both deodorant and talcum powder may simulate a small calcification. **localization (Andolina, Wentz, Ballinger)**

399. (D) The 45° oblique position is most useful in locating a lesion superiorly-inferiorly from the nipple. **localization (Andolina, Wentz, Ballinger)**

400. (B) The medial tissue is superimposed over the lateral region on the 45° oblique position. **localization (Andolina, Wentz, Ballinger)**

REFERENCES

Akesson, E., Loeb, J., Wilson-Pauwels, L. *Thompson's Core Textbook of Anatomy*, Philadelphia: J.B. Lippincott, 2nd ed., 1990.

American College of Radiology, *Mammography Quality Control Radiologic Technologist Manual*, Reston, VA: The American College of Radiology, 1990.

American Society of Radiologic Technologists, *Fundamentals of Mammography: The Quest for Quality Positioning Guidebook*, Albuquerque: The American Society of Radiologic Technologists, 1991.

Anderson, I., "Mammography in Clinical Practice," *Medical Radiography and Photography*, Rochester, NY: Eastman Kodak Co., Vol. 62, No. 2, 1986.

Andolina, V.F., Lille, S., Willison, K.M., *Mammographic Imaging: A Practical Guide*, Philadelphia: J.B. Lippincott, 1992.

Ballinger, P. W., *Merrill's Atlas of Radiographic Positions and Radiologic Procedures*, St. Louis: C.V. Mosby Co., 7th ed., Volume 3, 1991.

Bassett, L.W., Gold, R.H., *Mammography, Thermography, and Ultrasound in Breast Cancer Detection*, New York: Grune and Stratton, 1982.

Bassett, L.W., Gold, R.H., *Breast Cancer Detection: Mammography and Other Methods in Breast Imaging*, 2nd edition, Orlando: Grune and Stratton, Inc., 1987.

Bontrager, K., *Textbook of Radiographic Positioning and Related Anatomy*, St. Louis: C.V. Mosby Co., 1987.

Bushong, S., *Radiologic Science for Technologists*, St. Louis: C.V. Mosby Co., 4th ed., 1988.

Carlton, R., Adler, A.M., *Principles of Radiographic Imaging*, Albany: Delmar Publishers, 1992.

Cullinan, A.M., *Producing Quality Radiographs*, Philadelphia: J.B. Lippincott, 1987.

Curry, T.S., Dowdey, J.E., Murry, R.C., *Christensen's Physics of Diagnostic Radiology*, Philadelphia: Lea & Febiger Co., 4th ed., 1990.

Eklund, G.W., Busby, R.C., Miller, S.H., Job, J.S., "Improved Imaging of the Augmented Breast," *American Journal of Roentgenology*, 151: 469-473, 1988.

Egan, R.L., *Breast Imaging*, 3rd edition, Baltimore: University Park Press, 1984.

Eisenberg, R.L., Dennis, C.A., May, C.R., *Radiographic Positioning*, Boston: Little, Brown, and Company, 1989.

Fajardo, L.L., Westerman, B.R., "Mammography Equipment: Practical Considerations for the Radiologist," *Applied Radiology*, May, 12-15, 1990.

Feig, S., "Estimation of Radiation Risk from Screening Mammography: Recent Trends and Comparison with Expected Benefits," *Radiology*, Vo. 174, 638-647, 1990.

Gray, Joel E., Winkler, Norlin T., Stears, John, and Frank, Eugene D., *Quality Control in Diagnostic Imaging*, Baltimore: University Park Press, 1983.

Gurley, T.G., Callaway, W.J., *Introduction to Radiologic Technology*, 3rd edition, St. Louis: C.V. Mosby Co., 1992.

Hole, John W., Jr., *Human Anatomy and Physiology*, Dubuque: Wm. C. Brown Co., 2nd edition, 1981.

Long, Shirley M., *Handbook of Mammography*, 2nd edition, Edmonton, Alberta, Canada: Mammography Consulting Services/Convention graphics, 1990.*

Mitchell, G.W., Bassett, L.W., *The Female Breast and Its Disorders*, Baltimore: Williams and Wilkins, 1990.

NCRP Report No. 85, *Mammography: A User's Guide*, Bethesda, MD: National Council on Radiation Protection and Measurements, 1991.

Scanlon, E.F., "Breast Cancer," Chapter 13 from Holleb, A.I., Fink, D.J., Murphy, G.P., *American Cancer Society Textbook of Clinical Oncology*, Atlanta: American Cancer Society, 177-193, 1991.

Torres, L.S., *Basic Medical Techniques and Patient Care for Radiologic Technologists*, 3rd edition, Philadelphia: J.B. Lippincott Co., 1989.

U.S. Department of Health and Human Services, *The Breast Cancer Digest*, 2nd edition, Washington, D.C.: National Institutes of Health, Public Health Services, 1984.

Wentz, G., *Mammography for Radiologic Technologists*, New York: McGraw-Hill, 1992.

*This resource was designed to accompany the Mammography Correspondence Course of the Canadian Association of Medical Radiation Technologists. It has been privately published and is available from Mammography Consulting Services, 1024 82nd Street, Edmonton, Alberta, Canada T6K 1X6, phone 403-462-2615.

APPENDIX A
SIMULATED EXAMINATION 1 ANSWERS

1.	A	26.	A	51.	D	76.	C
2.	C	27.	D	52.	C	77.	C
3.	B	28.	D	53.	D	78.	A
4.	C	29.	B	54.	B	79.	A
5.	C	30.	C	55.	A	80.	B
6.	C	31.	D	56.	D	81.	C
7.	D	32.	C	57.	C	82.	B
8.	C	33.	B	58.	D	83.	B
9.	A	34.	A	59.	C	84.	B
10.	C	35.	A	60.	D	85.	D
11.	C	36.	D	61.	A	86.	B
12.	D	37.	A	62.	C	87.	A
13.	D	38.	C	63.	C	88.	B
14.	D	39.	B	64.	B	89.	D
15.	D	40.	D	65.	A	90.	A
16.	A	41.	D	66.	C	91.	B
17.	C	42.	B	67.	C	92.	B
18.	B	43.	C	68.	B	93.	A
19.	C	44.	D	69.	D	94.	A
20.	C	45.	A	70.	A	95.	C
21.	D	46.	B	71.	C	96.	B
22.	D	47.	A	72.	A	97.	C
23.	B	48.	A	73.	C	98.	C
24.	B	49.	C	74.	C	99.	C
25.	C	50.	A	75.	B	100.	A

APPENDIX B
SIMULATED EXAMINATION 2 ANSWERS

1.	B	26.	D	51.	D	76.	A
2.	B	27.	C	52.	D	77.	C
3.	B	28.	D	53.	A	78.	A
4.	A	29.	A	54.	D	79.	A
5.	D	30.	B	55.	B	80.	C
6.	A	31.	A	56.	B	81.	D
7.	D	32.	B	57.	B	82.	D
8.	C	33.	C	58.	A	83.	C
9.	B	34.	D	59.	D	84.	A
10.	C	35.	C	60.	C	85.	D
11.	D	36.	D	61.	D	86.	A
12.	D	37.	D	62.	B	87.	B
13.	B	38.	C	63.	C	88.	B
14.	A	39.	A	64.	B	89.	A
15.	B	40.	B	65.	D	90.	B
16.	C	41.	D	66.	B	91.	C
17.	A	42.	B	67.	A	92.	C
18.	A	43.	A	68.	A	93.	A
19.	C	44.	B	69.	C	94.	D
20.	D	45.	C	70.	A	95.	D
21.	C	46.	A	71.	B	96.	A
22.	D	47.	B	72.	B	97.	A
23.	A	48.	A	73.	D	98.	B
24.	C	49.	C	74.	C	99.	C
25.	A	50.	A	75.	C	100.	C

APPENDIX C
SIMULATED EXAMINATION 3 ANSWERS

1.	B	26.	A	51.	A	76.	A
2.	B	27.	B	52.	C	77.	D
3.	A	28.	C	53.	A	78.	A
4.	B	29.	B	54.	A	79.	B
5.	A	30.	D	55.	C	80.	D
6.	A	31.	D	56.	C	81.	A
7.	D	32.	A	57.	D	82.	C
8.	A	33.	B	58.	D	83.	B
9.	D	34.	C	59.	A	84.	C
10.	A	35.	D	60.	A	85.	A
11.	B	36.	B	61.	A	86.	C
12.	C	37.	C	62.	A	87.	B
13.	A	38.	D	63.	A	88.	D
14.	A	39.	B	64.	D	89.	B
15.	B	40.	B	65.	A	90.	A
16.	C	41.	A	66.	A	91.	B
17.	D	42.	D	67.	B	92.	D
18.	C	43.	D	68.	A	93.	A
19.	A	44.	B	69.	D	94.	C
20.	B	45.	B	70.	B	95.	A
21.	B	46.	C	71.	B	96.	B
22.	B	47.	D	72.	C	97.	B
23.	C	48.	C	73.	C	98.	A
24.	B	49.	C	74.	B	99.	B
25.	D	50.	B	75.	D	100.	C

APPENDIX D
SIMULATED EXAMINATION 4 ANSWERS

1.	A	26.	D	51.	B	76.	A
2.	D	27.	B	52.	D	77.	A
3.	B	28.	A	53.	A	78.	C
4.	D	29.	A	54.	C	79.	C
5.	A	30.	B	55.	A	80.	A
6.	A	31.	B	56.	B	81.	B
7.	C	32.	C	57.	A	82.	B
8.	D	33.	C	58.	A	83.	A
9.	D	34.	C	59.	A	84.	C
10.	D	35.	B	60.	C	85.	D
11.	A	36.	A	61.	D	86.	A
12.	D	37.	D	62.	D	87.	D
13.	C	38.	C	63.	A	88.	B
14.	D	39.	B	64.	B	89.	C
15.	B	40.	A	65.	B	90.	D
16.	D	41.	A	66.	D	91.	C
17.	C	42.	A	67.	B	92.	B
18.	A	43.	D	68.	A	93.	A
19.	D	44.	B	69.	C	94.	C
20.	C	45.	A	70.	B	95.	B
21.	D	46.	B	71.	C	96.	B
22.	D	47.	A	72.	B	97.	A
23.	A	48.	A	73.	A	98.	A
24.	B	49.	B	74.	D	99.	D
25.	B	50.	B	75.	A	100.	B

APPENDIX E
COMMON ABBREVIATIONS AND ACRONYMS

AT   axillary tail (oblique lateral or Cleopatra)
CC   craniocaudal
CV   cleavage
EDPT extended developer processing time
FB   caudocranial (from below)
L   left
LM   90° lateromedial
LMO   lateromedial oblique
M   magnification
ML   90° mediolateral
MLO   mediolateral oblique
R   right
RL   rolled lateral
RM   rolled medial
SIO   superolateral to inferomedial oblique
TAN   tangential
XCCL exaggerated craniocaudal